THE MIRACLE BALL METHOD

for Chronic Lower Back Pain

BY ELAINE PETRONE

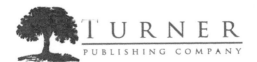

TURNER
PUBLISHING COMPANY

Turner Publishing Company
Nashville, Tennessee
www.turnerpublishing.com

The Miracle Ball Method for Chronic Lower Back Pain
Copyright © 2021 Elaine Petrone

Book design by Stacy Wakefield Forte
Photography by Gary Spector
Library of Congress Cataloging-in-Publication Data

Names: Petrone, Elaine, author.
Title: The miracle ball method for chronic lower back pain / Elaine
   Petrone.
Description: First edition. | Nashville : Turner Publishing Company, 2021.
Identifiers: LCCN 2021021837 (print) | LCCN 2021021838 (ebook) ISBN   9781684425976 (paperback) | ISBN 9781684425990 (ebook)
Subjects: LCSH: Backache--Exercise therapy. | Stress management. Chronic   pain--Alternative treatment.
Classification:
LCC RD771.B217 P4745 2021 (print) LCC RD771.B217   (ebook) DDC 617.5/64062--dc23
LC record available at https://lccn.loc.gov/2021021837
LC ebook record available at https://lccn.loc.gov/2021021838

Printed in the United States of America

Disclaimer: The special needs limitations and responses of each individual cannot be anticipated. The Miracle Ball Method is not intended for the purpose of diagnosing or as a substitute for medical attention.

This book is for all my students over the years that have joined me on this journey.

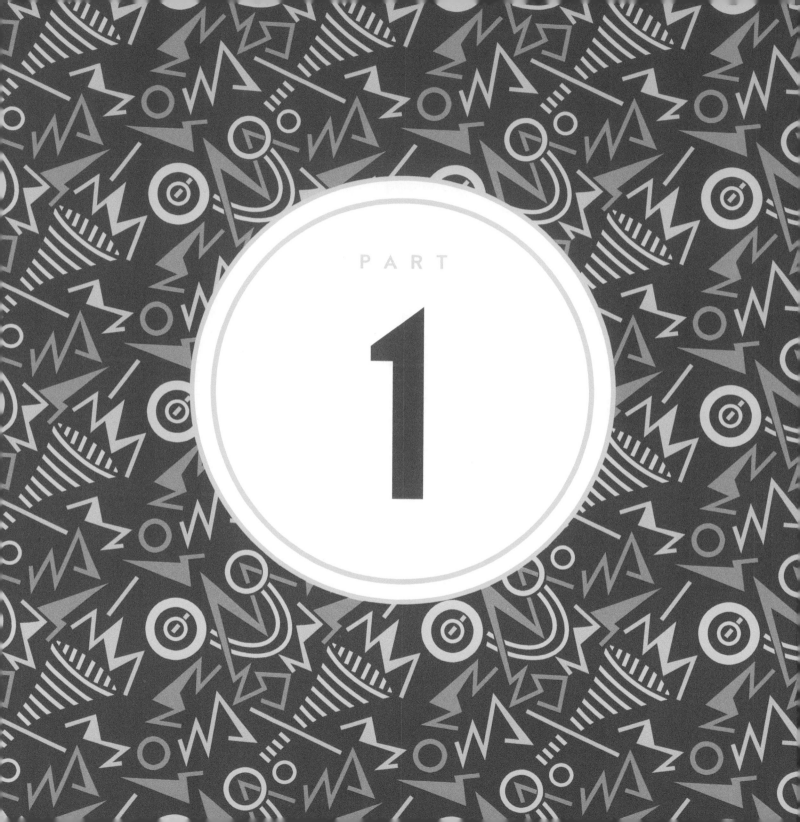

PART

1

WELCOME TO the Miracle Ball Method. This is a book for people with chronic lower back pain that seems to run their lives, people who have tried everything and lost confidence and need answers. Eighty percent of Americans will experience back pain in their lifetimes and it is on the rise. Nine out of ten patients never know what caused it because there are many contributing factors. Americans spend at least 50 billion dollars a year to treat back pain. Approximately half of the people who experience an initial episode of back pain will have reoccurrences and some become chronic.

I was where you are. Back pain can happen at any age, and my pain relief journey began when I was nineteen. After much trial and error and no relief, I discovered I was going in completely the wrong direction. I did everything I was told and more. But sooner or later the pain always returned. The treatments today are not that much different than they were then, there are just more of them now.

After teaching in hospitals for over 25 years, where those who attended classes had a wide range of backgrounds including health professionals, I learned that the biggest mistake people make is relying completely on someone else to heal them. They look outside of their own body to find relief. They are looking elsewhere, anyplace other than themselves for answers. It's as if we are saying to ourselves, my body is doing something wrong, and I need to fix it. It needs a cure. But we know back pain isn't a disease. We have to reframe/change the dialogue. Most of us assume that we "control" our body. If you have ever had chronic lower back pain, you probably know much of the frustration is feeling out of control. "Why does this return? I have tried everything."

The Miracle in this Method is your body can and

will give you the solutions to relieve your pain and help you to move freely without fear. The missing link is we don't control our bodies. It's somewhat of a partnership, if you think about it. You are constantly receiving information from your body. We are familiar with our five senses–seeing, hearing, tasting, touch and smell–but few of us understand how we can develop our kinesthetic sense just like any of the five senses. The amazing thing about the muscular skeletal system is that it is extremely adaptable. We are training it inadvertently all the time. Unfortunately, our training is limited because of how complicated pain is. We avoid a lot of the movements, and directions that would give us relief and make us much stronger.

With the Miracle Ball Method, you will use the innate sense our body has to adjust and align, thus taking the stress off your lower back. Because you are in this partnership with your body, you will guide it with some simple directions as we move forward in this book.

My moment was when I actually noticed my body do something without me….. and I had relief. It was a moment. But that moment made me realize I had no idea what was causing this pain, and I had to go in this direction. The Method works; it only doesn't work if you don't do it!

There are layers and layers of history ruling our body. There are stresses, injuries, and illnesses that have left their marks. Unraveling these layers of twisted muscle tension is possible and essential. Without it, we are going in a direction that continuously debilitates us.

Chronic pain is the result of what we do with our whole body. Just as a detective puts together evidence, you can sift through your body's clues to learn what you may be unknowingly doing to contribute to your ongoing discomfort. When you discover how to do this—which is what I'll teach you in this book—you'll find that your body can actually give you feedback, and ultimately, solutions.

RELAX, RELEASE, AND LET GO

The Miracle Ball Method is an innovative approach that reduces excess muscle tension, which in turn will relieve your pain, reshape your body, and reduce stress. The Method is relearning a system in your own body that holds the answers for so many of the everyday conditions we live with that cause discomfort.

The Miracle Ball Method is not an exercise program. The miracle is in your own body, as are the answers for so many of the conditions we live with that cause discomfort. My students named the Method, and it just stuck over time. At the end of class, they would consistently look puzzled, especially if they came in with nagging lower back pain, a tight neck, or tense shoulder muscles. Then they would report with a confused look on their face, "It's gone." They were so confused because the directions I had given them were so simple. They felt like they had done nothing. The directions leave room for the body to respond and for your nervous system to reorganize. It knows what to do. This is what you will be learning. The directions are simple; people are complicated.

What makes the Miracle Ball Method different is it gives you the tools to know your body in a much deeper way than many of us have ever thought about. You will discover that your body has its own ability to realign and recover from chronic pain, injury, illness, and the stressors of everyday life. But first we have to develop or retrain our ability to sense or "feel" our body more fully.

Beware of mistaking the Miracle Ball Method for release, relax, or let-go methods. Although these may be the results we get with the Miracle Ball Method, those are not the directions. Having strong, supportive muscles that do not hurt and are not stiff is our goal.

Many of us love relaxation and letting go. But letting go of the body sometimes seriously disconnects us from feeling the body. Instead of trying to release or relax all tension, think of tension as what connects all parts of our body and as essential to improving our breath.

Most exercise programs work the muscles, but it is the nervous system, the underlying connection to the muscles, that can transform your body. Our nervous system is available to us, and it has the ability to transform our mind and body at any age.

We need to understand that we are capable of being extremely strong even after injuries. Even conditions that we have lived with for a lifetime can change. But we will have to redevelop our kinesthetic sense—

Kinesthetic: Learning through feeling, such as a sense of body position, muscle movement, and weight as felt through nerve endings. An example of kinesthetic is the nature of a workout in gym class. An example of kinesthetic is learning to ride a bike by actually getting on the bike and riding, not just hearing about how to do it.

in other words, "feel" our bodies. Otherwise our bodies have no new information to use, and we continue to be stuck in our habits of movement that we are not even aware of. Most of us have not harnessed the power of our ability to use the kinesthetic sense. By developing this ability, our nervous system can then make the changes needed to relieve pain, move more freely, and alleviate much of the personal stress associated with pain.

Most of us are familiar with exercise, medical treatments, or relaxation. All of these are things we do to our body. The Miracle Ball Method is your body doing it. Your body is the instrument, and the Method is how you tune it up. This prepares you and improves any endeavor or activity you do. Your whole self is stimulated.

The directions for the Method are very specific. Some of my students have described them as counterintuitive. We think that since we hurt a lot, we need a complicated solution. I have learned through my own experience with chronic lower back pain—and teaching hundreds of thousands of others, including health professionals—that once the body has this experience, the pain is relieved.

MYTHS AND MISUNDERSTANDINGS

Because many of us spend our lives trying to avoid another back spasm or control our level of pain, we are vigilant all the time. There are many things we are told to do and many things we think we have to avoid. Maybe you exercise tirelessly to make the pain go away or take medication constantly. Some of us go to therapy for years. Don't mistake this for "the pain is all in my head." It's not. It's all connected.

Here are some of the beliefs and worries we often cling to as we go through life with chronic lower back pain. Do you identify with any of these?

IS YOUR BODY STUCK?

There are many different kinds of pain. Pain is difficult to address as simply pain, like one lump. With chronic pain its difficult to get results because when people say *pain*, they don't realize there are different components at work. You have to address these different aspects of pain. This will make it easier to then break it down and get relief. Pain comprises your thoughts, muscle tension, and breathing. These are interconnected. Some of us are more affected by our thoughts, whereas others are more vigilant for physical sensations. Our breathing responds to both instantly. When we break it down, we can begin to notice what we might be doing that triggers more pain.

Chronic lower back pain is the result of what I will refer to as your "stuck body." By "stuck," I mean that your muscles get stiff and tight in postures and positions unique to you—often without you even realizing it. The result is excess muscle tension. This tension affects your breathing and your ability to improve long term, even with all the treatments you may have tried. When you are stuck you have to break down the feeling into three parts, the thoughts—what information you are telling yourself about your problem—how your muscles actually feel, and your breathing.

I reduce excess muscle tension using a language that your body can respond to. I have found by reducing the excess muscle tension your body is able to make adjustments and realign. It relearns what you once did easily. You will no longer be stuck. You will find balance and flexibility.

The Miracle Ball Method is not exercise. The Miracle Ball Method will give you specific directions to access your nervous system, the underlying connection that allows all your parts to work together to make movement. Your body is designed to realign and adjust on a daily basis. Once you understand how to communicate with your body, you will discover how to let your body make adjustments.

You will also discover that you have two very clear roads. One leads to repeating the movements of your stuck body, and the other leads to an ability most of us have and simply never use that allows your body to unwind and recover. The Method is very clear, easy to do, and somewhat miraculous to feel. It is also a learning process, or a re-learning process. But it is a learning process that anyone can do, like riding a bike or learning to cook.

Imagine having the active lifestyle you crave and the added benefits of a rewarding mind–body connection—all achieved by you and the Miracle Ball Method.

+ You have to know your stuck body, and what part you play in that.

+ When you feel better, you have to acknowledge physically what's changed. It's different for every person.

+ Prevent yourself from returning to the stuck body by replacing it with something you've learned, and move freely without pain.

UNLEARNING OUR HABITS OF MOVEMENT?

Exercises, treatments, and surgery many times don't work because we are missing the elephant in the room: our bodies are ruled by our unique physical habits of movement. Your habits are the result of your history of injury, alignment, and stress. If we are not aware of these habits, we may feel good for a while, but then we always return to our stuck body.

That is why so many things like trying to ease tension with a tennis ball or a foam roller work for a while but then pain returns. Many of us use the same amount of effort in the muscles that are already overworked even while we seek relief. Our habits are still very much alive. When we stop rubbing and pressing, the circulation leaves the muscles and we feel the same discomfort.

You cannot get back to the great feeling you had after your medical treatments, because you don't know what your body did to get there. In other words, something physically changed after your treatment.

We don't understand exactly what that is. We also don't know what changes physically after the treatment to make us hurt again.

Without that missing link, we will always return to the stuck body or habit of movement. You have trained your body to move and breathe certain ways. It gets reinforced over time.

Even if we are aware of our habits, we must go deeper. I may be aware there is a piano in the room, and I may be able to play a few songs. But does that mean I really know the instrument? Think of your body like this instrument. Your body has a kinesthetic sense to help you feel movement. Without rediscovering the ability to feel more parts of the body through this kinesthetic sense, you remain stuck.

Throughout this book, I will simply use the word

"feel" rather than "sense" when referring to the nervous system. The Method is designed to increase feeling. You will use cues that your body will understand to guide yourself, and your brain will begin to work with this feedback from all these new very specific feelings.

It is very individual. You may be doing something very specific with your hips, your breathing, your shoulders that are your unique self. When you start feeling that, your brain knows what to do with that information. Even better, you can then begin to do whatever activity you enjoy but with this awareness that "Oh, I don't need to use those muscles like that; I can do it this way." Remember, we learned how to walk from experimenting, from trial and error. Your brain processed specifically what worked and what didn't until you were happily upright. If you had to stop and analyze each movement or understand anatomy, you would have never gotten out of the crib. It was spontaneous. (Though some days were more successful than others, I would imagine.)

As adults, we are not so confident. Back pain can be so disturbing that it takes our confidence away. We begin to look for answers, and many health professionals will make you more afraid to move, which activates more anxiety. Remember, pain is a combination of our thoughts, our muscle tension, and our breathing.

THE CYCLE OF PAIN

While we all have similar parts, each of our bodies is a unique machine, one that each of us maneuvers differently, creating conditions that often result in what

I call the "cycle of pain." Being trapped in the pain and discomfort of this cycle causes us to hold our breath for relief, which only leads to more pain and discomfort, which then leads to potentially elevated stress levels, which then can lead to chronic situations . . . and round and round we go.

The stuck body requires a tremendous amount of excess muscle tension. Think of squeezing a tennis ball very hard, then continuing to do that for hours or days. Eventually you would feel pain in many parts of your body. You may not even know how to let go of the tennis ball, your muscles will have gotten so tight.

This excess tension in our stuck body can come from three sources: an accident or sports injury; stress from daily life or more complicated issues; and alignment issues, such as scoliosis or poor posture. You may have one of these sources or, as I did, all three.

No matter the origin of the tension, your muscles respond in the cycle of pain. For instance, you may feel the origin is in your back. But holding your muscles very stiffly results in shallow breathing. Poor breathing habits result in more stress. Elevated stress makes our muscles tighten. The cycle goes around and around and we are caught in this loop.

Chronic lower back pain is the result of the cycle of pain. But each person's cycle is a bit different. You may be more inclined to heighten your fears and anxieties, your stress. Another person may be more focused on holding their breath or perhaps stiffening their muscles when they move.

I have found as we ease the excess muscle ten-

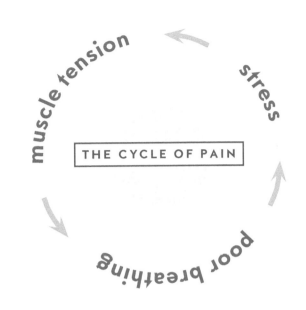

muscle tension

stress

THE CYCLE OF PAIN

poor breathing

sion our bodies can begin to experience relief. You will begin to distinguish each part of the cycle more easily. As you affect one, the others naturally benefit. You begin to move away from being stuck until you are free from the pain. Believe it or not, pain is not a bad thing. Pain is a warning signal.

Even lower back pain, which is as painful as can be or sometimes just relentlessly nagging and uncomfortable, is telling us something, a way that the body is giving direction. Because we think of pain as one thing "pain" and we don't understand it, we don't realize it actually is giving us the directions how to get out of it.

Most of us don't think our body has the ability to tell us things, but think about it. If you put your hand on a hot stove, your sense of touch is going to cause

you to pull away quickly. If you taste something bad, you spit it out. If you hear a terrible noise, you turn around to investigate. With our body, our kinesthetic sense is telling us we are moving in a way that is giving us pain. We don't listen because we are fearful of the pain. It must be bad. We want to change it. We don't recognize that we have options. The body can be very specific, but when pain comes with fear, most people want a way out.

By developing this kinesthetic sense through the easy directions in this book, you will find that your pain will lessen and, most importantly, lead you to where you need to go. Over time, you will gain confidence that your body knows what to do. It won't be an accident or a feeling of "What do I do now?" You will know what to do.

Back pain can feel anywhere from mildly uncomfortable to debilitating. I will lay out different levels of pain, so when you go through the book and begin the Method, start with whichever section that aligns with your level of chronic lower back pain.

Don't get discouraged. If you start playing the guitar, learning to cook, going to medical school, or training yourself to fix cars, you expect a lot of trial and error. You might even struggle with painful calluses on your fingers from playing the guitar or headaches and eyestrain from being at the computer. But you continue and reap the benefits of your efforts. With back pain, there is a mystery that makes many of us worry:

"What will happen?

What if it doesn't go away?"

"Tom up the street has had back pain along with three surgeries."

"Rosemary has scoliosis and suffers with sciatic pain. What if my pain never goes away, like hers?"

We get trapped by these thoughts. None of these worries apply, because no two people are alike. We all have different fingerprints, and we all live in our bodies differently. We have different lifestyles, behaviors, history, likes and dislikes, and we all respond to pain differently. Give yourself some time to follow the directions and let your body respond.

MY EXPERIENCE

I had pain that eventually left me bedridden. I was afraid to move. I crawled to the bathroom and cried a lot. There was pain from the top of my head to my toes at times. Numbness moved through my body. My left leg got weaker and weaker. Despite many doctors, nothing made sense.

I learned that the pain started in one place, but my thoughts and experiences at the time made me very anxious, and that was exacerbating my pain. That is why it's very hard to just "cure" the pain. My fears kept me in bed, and perhaps for a couple of days that would have been fine. But I stayed there much longer. Then when I began to move, I had become so deconditioned, I was feeling pain from many sources: my anxiety, and my muscles had become weakened over time. The lack of support to move again, and the original problem.

As I began to get relief from my aching back after combining many different approaches, I started to learn that it was my body making changes. That realization took me in a completely unexpected direction. Although I had relief, my biggest concern was that I didn't want it to be an accident. I didn't want the relief to be short lived. I didn't want to be afraid to pick something up, bend over, or dance again (although everyone told me dancing again was out of the question anyway).

I did get relief after I began to understand the directions my body was sending. The body will send you information so you can relearn what feels good and move away from what doesn't. We have to move in order to understand the body. But most people with chronic pain think it's best not to move. Just as I hope you will learn in this book, as I reduced excess muscle tension, I learned my body wasn't just relaxing. It was realigning.

I didn't just stand up and go on with my day after using the Method. I noticed I walked differently. Most importantly, I breathed, which had never been something that came easily to me. As I finally got relief, I wanted to tell others. In fact, it felt like I was drafted into a world of body work where I had never planned on going. But I had to tell people. It became a mission more than a method. If I could improve, anyone could improve.

Somehow, I met doctors who themselves had chronic pain and who asked for my help; so did my next-door neighbors. Forty years later, here I am. There have been millions of books sold, and the Miracle Ball Method has helped people around the world. I sincerely hope it will do the same for you. You can also go to my website (www.miracleballmethod.com) for information and free webinars. Take classes online and don't ever be discouraged.

YOUR CHECK-IN

Do you have a stuck body—a place or position that you seem to fight with, or just never move out of?

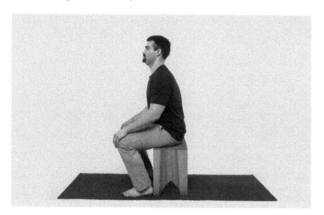

Before we move on, maybe you would like to give yourself a quick assessment. See what you notice when you bring attention to your body. This should only take about fifteen seconds. No need to get complicated. A quick example of how easily you can use your kinesthetic sense. You can begin sitting either on the floor or a chair.

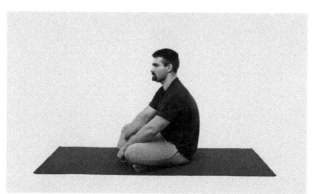

Because pain is not pleasurable, many of us want to avoid taking this step. We just want to be rid of the pain. I have found from talking to so many people that many of us have the ability to notice what is wrong with us in detail, but we think it isn't helpful. In fact, we just need to learn to use that information. That is the kinesthetic sense. When we acknowledge it, we can take control of our progress by using it.

Do you see two people here that stand, look, exactly the same?

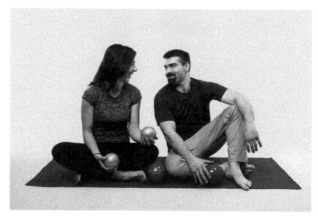

ASSESSING THE SIGNALS

Describe exactly what you feel. Avoid emotions or what others have told you. Describe your body as if you were describing it to an alien who doesn't have a body. What does it feel like? You can do this standing, sitting, or lying down. I have found most people have a really good sense of their body but have to be encouraged that they will find answers in what they notice.

As you go through this initial assessment, you will have many physical feelings related to the cycle of pain. Muscle tightness, breathing, and maybe thoughts or stresses will be front and center.

Can you break it down? Each of the categories I have mentioned can be different. For some, muscle tension is predominant. For others, it's the holding of the breath or the thoughts that are overwhelming. Each one contributes to the other, and it's hard to change until we break it down with the Method. The good news is there are no right and wrong answers.

Here are some examples of how people describe their first assessment of the stuck body. Try to include what you notice physically and any sense of breathing. Or are you simply focused on your thoughts?

In the future, we will simply call this the Check-In, and it takes about fifteen seconds during your day to notice any of the pieces of the cycle of pain. You can take this ability with you anywhere, because it's as simple as using any of your five senses.

+ My chest muscles are tight (physical)

+ My lower back hurts (physical)

+ I can't feel my breathing (breathing)

+ My shoulders are rounded forward (physical)

+ I am anxious (thought)

+ I want to lie down (thought)

GETTING STARTED

Chapter 1 will go over basic set up to easily do the Method. Chapter 2 will include some terms, or the language that will communicate to your physical body. Chapter 3 will include key areas that are essential to have a lower back free from chronic pain. Before you begin, see the highlighted area below. Although there are probably as many experiences with pain as there are different kinds of people, to use this book most effectively, see which category most describes you at this time. Whichever category you choose, there will be suggestions through the different ball placements and Whole Body Moves as to what might work best. As time goes on, you will improve and can gradually decide where you might want to go next in the book as far as ball placements and Whole Body Moves. Breathing at any time is always beneficial. ESSENTIAL. Breathing is what brings feeling into the muscles and allows your nervous system to use that information. Without this connection to your personal way of breathing, we miss a key link to long term change.

Many people with chronic pain unknowingly repeat patterns of movement and breathing that keep them stuck. The less you move, the less you will move and the more pain you will have. You may have sought relief through yoga, massage, or chiropractic. Although many of these are harmless and could be helpful, they are often only a temporary fix. If you are still fighting with the underlying habits that you unknowingly have, you remain stuck in a painful position.

Be open minded. Our thoughts are seamlessly aligned with our musculature and our breathing. If we are fearful and convinced that we will never move freely again or that our pain will be constant, our muscles will respond to that fear and aggravate what we are feeling by tightening up further. Let's get started!

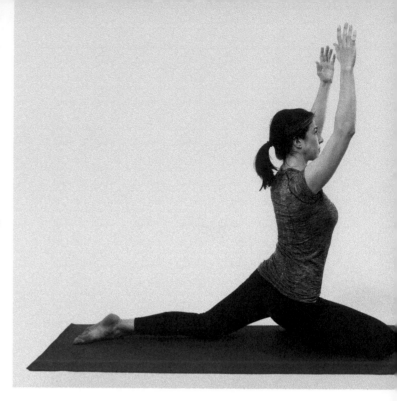

+ Deep breathing will solve it.

+ I do yoga and tai chi and my back and hip still hurt.

+ I shouldn't bend over or arch.

+ I coughed and my back went out, so I am afraid.

+ A strong core will stop my pain.

+ I need to be more relaxed.

+ I need to get rid of the stress in my life.

+ I need to be careful when I move.

+ I shouldn't move when I have pain.

+ I should avoid exercise.

+ Relax, release, and let-go body methods heal the back.

CHAPTER ONE

HOW TO USE THIS BOOK

THE BOOK IS divided into three parts. Part 1 is to get you familiar with the Method, as it's quite different from other body Methods. It will describe some of the equipment, key areas of the body, as well as some of the familiar terms to use or "cues" that your body will respond to. You will get introduced to some basics on breathing. This fundamental understanding is not included in many other health and fitness practices because it is not in their training. But by learning how to use and improve your kinesthetic sense, all other body methods will be more effective.

In part 2, you will begin to do the Method. Get used to the easygoing back-and-forth with your body using the directions. You will use the balls, and what I call Whole Body Moves to transform your body. Combined, the balls and your breathing create a brain–body connection. That brain–body connection allows the nervous system to give you new information.

That information helps you relearn what your body did naturally years ago.

Part 3 will help you take what you're learning into your everyday life. It will answer some commonly asked questions and advise you how to use the Method throughout your day. You will become familiar with the idea that what you sensed on the balls, is just as easy to apply to your tennis game, or a walk in the park.

You do not have to do every breathing technique and ball placement. It would be best to pick one and let your body respond. Less is more.

Since this is not exercise, the more familiar you get with the easygoing back-and-forth directions, the more responsive you will be. They are not difficult, and yet students constantly stray from them. I am told they are somewhat counterintuitive. But they are tried and true. When I bring people back to the directions, they get the *aha* moment.

As you use the Method, it's likely you'll experience many new physical feelings, which will begin to replace the habits that are hurting you. Especially if you have had an illness or injury, along with lower back pain, you might fear certain physical sensations and begin to mislabel them. Try not to fear these new feelings. I have worked with thousands of people with chronic pain. Often as soon as they get an inkling of feeling in the body, their fight-or-flight system comes into play, and they freeze. They are convinced these feelings will begin to set off their pain again. As a result, they get weaker and weaker. Allow your body to respond.

Our thoughts and physical feelings are intertwined. Make the process easygoing; the terms you will read about next will help you to develop more confidence in your body. You should not have pain while doing the Method.

The Method will help reduce excess muscle tension. Excess muscle tension tightens our muscles, which affects our ability to breathe easily, which causes more stress. It becomes a cycle. You may feel stressed from an injury, then begin to hold your breath, and then feel more pain.

I use the phrase "excess tension" because I want to be clear. Tension is important; we want good muscle tension. There are too many misunderstandings where people are taught that "relax" or "release" means having no tension. Lack of tension is dangerous and promotes weakness in the body. We do not want to cultivate weakness but regain a strong foundation in our muscles and bones, the underlying support of our nervous system.

Gradually allow yourself to change. As you release excess muscle tension, you will notice changes not just in your muscles but also in your breathing and mental outlook. Acknowledge these changes. In the next chapter, you'll learn some terms so you can easily navigate through this new territory.

Even though you may feel this is a lot, it's actually just different. The Check-In really is fifteen to twenty seconds (see page 24). This is how you will build your vocabulary of feelings, just like going to a country with a foreign language. You start out with one word. Then you are speaking in sentences. Use the Check-In to get some sense of what you feel, and over time you will notice your body has thousands of different feelings.

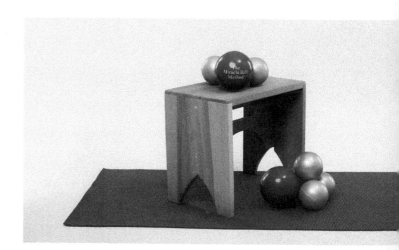

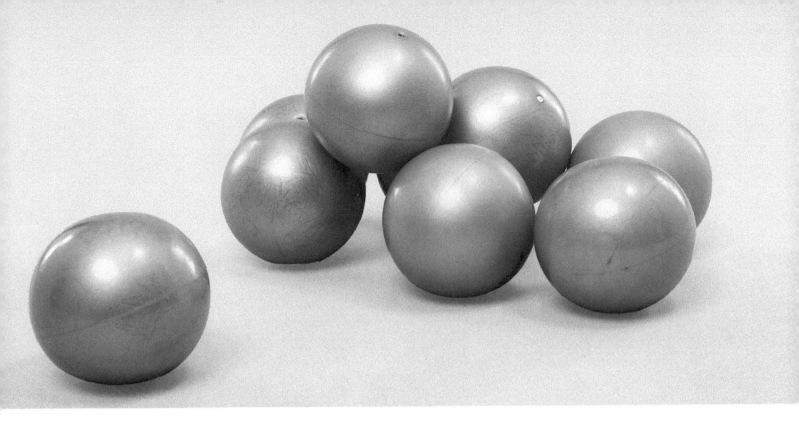

FREQUENTLY ASKED QUESTIONS

HOW DO I BEGIN? Begin with the Check-In (p. 24). You can start your Check-In either sitting or standing. The best thing to do is to find a bench or a chair of a good height and use that. Try to leave the phones off.

WHAT EQUIPMENT DO I NEED? Aside from a bench or chair, you'll need a mat or blankets for working on the floor. Since you might have a limited amount of time for how long you do your Check-In or hold each move, a clock within view might be handy. And of course, you'll need the Miracle Balls! If you do not have the balls, go to miracleballmethod.com/shop to order. Also on the website is a video to show you how to inflate or deflate using the valve provided in each ball. You can adjust the amount of air to meet your needs. There should be no pain when you're using the balls.

DO I NEED A SPECIAL PLACE IN MY HOUSE? At first, you'll benefit from finding a room with as few distractions as possible. After you fully understand the directions, you can do them pretty much anywhere. I used to have the balls in my children's bedroom. While they were toddlers, they simply wanted me in the room. I was on the floor with them. They thought

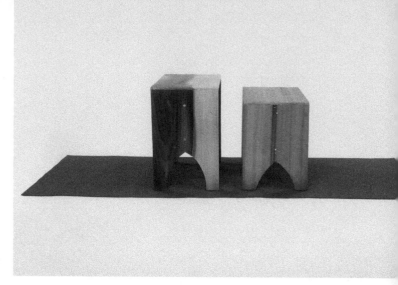

that was fun. But while they had their sticker books or Legos, I was making my _sss_ sound (see chapter 4) and doing my ball placements (see chapter 5). It was wonderful. I was a very calm mom at those times.

WHAT SHOULD I WEAR? Ideally, you want to have flexibility around your waistline so your diaphragmatic muscle is free to move. If you don't have time to change into more comfortable clothing, tight jeans need to be unbuttoned and unzipped. Tops that are too tight around your neck or chest need to be loosened.

Since you want to feel the movement of your body, loose clothing can be a disadvantage. I once had a ballet teacher who told us to wear headbands so we'd feel where our head was. To that I would add, wear Spandex or clothing that hugs you a bit so you can feel the muscles working under them.

MUST I LIE ON THE FLOOR? You have several options. The best place is on the floor if you are able to get up and down easily. If this is difficult, you can use your bench or chair to guide you down to the floor. But do not risk falling to the floor in a free fall and hope you land okay. Be logical; use your upper body strength and a gradual step-down approach. Have soft surfaces under you that don't slide. Some of the most strengthening exercises are getting up and down off the floor. If starting on a bed is best for you, do that. A firm mattress is best.

HOW LONG DOES IT TAKE TO FEEL BETTER? Just as with learning anything else, you can never tell how long it will take. Take your time and enjoy the process. Some people notice relief immediately. As you improve, you may find that when you don't do the Method you return to your habits. That is a way for your body to really sense what it is that makes you stuck. Remember, you are learning as much from what hurts as from what is helping.

SHOULD I STOP MY OTHER TREATMENTS? Learning and gaining benefit from different treatments is all good. Do not stop your other treatments unless you feel they are having a negative effect. If you do feel your treatments are not working, and they are with a health professional, express that. Having worked with doctors and many health professionals for years, I saw that they all appreciated that those who did the Method could communicate much more clearly about their experiences. In the end, you are building the ability to sense and thus move more and more of your body, to be stronger, and prevent back pain from returning.

HOW DO I FIND MY STUCK BODY? Use the Check-In to help you notice where you are stuck, holding your breath, or maintaining excess muscle tension. You can do it anywhere or anytime—standing in your kitchen, at a restaurant, at your desk. Sometimes you may notice you just want to stretch it or move it and it won't go where you want to. The stuckness may come and go. When you are under stress, you may feel it more easily. Our bodies return to familiar habits in times of worry and anxiety.

IT HURTS WHEN I MOVE; SHOULD I AVOID THAT MOVEMENT? Chronic lower back pain sets us up in a scenario where we begin to watch everything about the way we move. Sometimes we are afraid of movement because of past pain. But we have to move in order to improve. Use the Method to begin that journey again and change the negative dialogue. You will not always hurt when you move. There are reasons now why you do. Everything is trial and error. Although experience will give you a lot more success, there are always those times when you do something that doesn't work out. When that happens, just go back to the ball placements and breathe. Your body already has more experience at that point. Listen to the warning signals.

If you are not ready to do something, don't do it right now. But it doesn't mean you will never do that movement again.

WHAT TO EXPECT AFTER A FEW WEEKS OF MIRACLE BALL METHOD PRACTICE

Practice the Method two to three times a week. Once you are more experienced, having explored the breathing, ball placements, and Whole Body Moves, your sense of how you "feel" physically will be improved. You will be able to identify different parts of your body rather than just being jumbled up like a lump.

Once you understand how to use your kinesthetic sense, you will have more ability to move and breathe easier. As you learn the Method, you will realize throughout your day that you have options to move differently. As you begin to notice the way you carry yourself—and the way others carry themselves—it will become apparent that some adjustments are very easy and extremely beneficial.

Emotional and negative thoughts can make this difficult for many. We just simply don't believe we can move easily again or feel better. Many of us are cautiously optimistic. I know that the fear can make getting started difficult. But do it anyway. It's better to have a thousand wrong movements than one stuck movement you never stop doing.

Remember, your body does not want the back pain. Pain is a signal. You just haven't given it the options until now. It knows what to do. This is something over the next few months you will get better and better at.

CHAPTER TWO

MIRACLE BALL BASIC TERMS

BEFORE YOU CAN move on to how to feel better and address areas where you have pain, you will need to become proficient in Miracle Ball basic language. These are simple terms that describe how to encourage that brain–body connection. The actions that these terms define are easy to do but somewhat counterintuitive. Learn these basic terms and you are well on your way.

We begin with a **CHECK-IN**—something you can and will use easily throughout your daily life. The Check-In is simple observation of the three parts of pain: the muscle tension, the breath, and the thoughts. The more you feel, the more freely you will move. For example, the lower body, or core, is part of our center of gravity. These muscles can become twisted and clenched. (Think of gridlock at an intersection or a knot in your shoelace that seems impossible to loosen.) As you simply observe, your brain–body connection

goes to work. The clenching will gradually ease up as you include what you have learned, are you stuck or "holding" those muscles tightly? Are you holding your breath? You can't change what you don't feel.

Your **BODY DIALOGUE** is an unconscious communication between brain and body, moment to moment, throughout our lives. We usually don't have to think about getting out of a chair or how to climb stairs. We just move. When we have chronic lower back pain, we often do begin to think before each movement. We can become anxious, and we can activate a cycle of negative thoughts in a moment. Being aware of that is essential. Relearning to trust our body again is an important result of giving it a chance to respond. That is part of the dialogue.

The **BODY FORMULA** is your cues: the physical experiences of weight and the breath. These are the only two cues you really need to remember to reduce excess muscle tension.

Have you ever tried to stand up straight and noticed shortly after that your posture returns to its habit? We keep trying, but the body doesn't respond to such commands long term, if at all. The reason is that they are isolated thoughts that are not connected to real, physical feelings in the body. The good news is bodies are very adaptable. They just need the right directions. The Body Formula is using the weight of our different body parts, using the breath. If you remember nothing else, remember the feeling of the weight of your body and your breathing.

THE CHECK-IN

The Check-In is simply observing what you feel in your physical body at this point in time. Don't confuse it with what you like about your body or what you think you should do. Just make simple physical observations by checking in with your physical body.

People always tell me they couldn't practice because they were so overwhelmed by their backache or a worry they were having in their life. That is exactly when you do want to practice. Don't try to relax first.

There is a "transition" period, but your body will help to direct you as you calmly direct yourself back to noticing your body. Then begin with whatever ball placement, breathing, or Whole Body Moves you are planning.

Thoughts are of course different from the physical body. But they influence each other greatly and are completely intertwined. You really cannot stop your thoughts, but you can remind yourself, if your thoughts take you on a wild goose chase far from what you are doing, to go back to your physical feelings. Eventually your physical body will align with your thoughts more easily. Do not wait to do the Method until your thoughts are calm.

DOING A CHECK-IN

Feeling your body at the beginning of your session gives you a benchmark to compare with the changes by the end of the session. This specificity, of anything you notice about your physical body, activates the communication with your nervous system. It becomes your language to communicate with your body.

Lie down on the floor. If that is difficult, you can use a mat over a carpet or, if you are member of a gym, lie on a stretching table. You can also practice in bed on a firm mattress. A firm surface allows you to get a sense of your shape. You can also perform a Check-In while sitting on a hard bench or chair. Check in lying down.

Close your eyes. Take fifteen to twenty seconds and notice anything that might describe your posture and position to someone else who doesn't feel your body. Here are some initial descriptions some of my students have used when describing their physical body:

If lying down?

+ My lower back is off the floor.

+ My head is not resting, and my shoulders

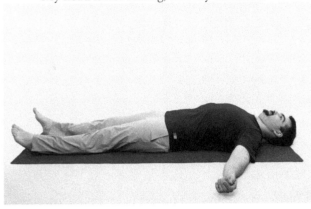

feel stiff.

+ My left hip feels higher than my right.

+ My neck feels shorter on the left side, and my chin is jutting forward.

+ Breathing is filling up the front of my upper chest.

+ My breathing is shallow.

These next observations are less specific about how the body is sitting, and more an emotional response:

+ My low back is tight, and I'm tired.

+ My right shoulder hurts.

+ I am very anxious and annoyed by this, and I want to lie down.

Thoughts about your body like "I am very uncomfortable" or "My lower back hurts" reinforce the problem but don't give your body direction. So break it down and be specific; notice where your breath is and what sensations stand out.

You don't have to feel good. You don't have to relax or have "good" posture. Lie normally and describe what you notice about your position and where you might feel your breathing. If you feel nothing, that's not uncommon. You will, in time. Knowing the difference between feeling nothing and forcing good posture or giving unhelpful answers deserves applause.

Here are some more specific things you may sense while resting on the floor:

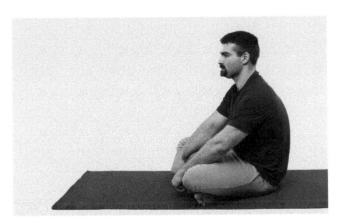

+ Notice the parts of your body that are resting comfortably on the floor.

+ Does one part of your body stand out as lifted off the floor (your lower back, the back of your neck, the back of your knees, your shoulders)?

+ Do you prefer your knees bent?

+ What part of your arms rest on the floor?

+ Where do you rest your head?

+ Is your chin tilted up or down?

Whatever you feel is perfect! It's not what you feel that activates your body's ability to make adjustments; it's that you feel, period. The more specifically you feel things, the better. Remember, what we lack is feeling because of all the excess muscle tension.

Many of us feel very little in the beginning. When I began this practice at age nineteen, no one had ever asked me what I felt. I thought feelings were more about my thoughts. But then I realized there were many physical feelings happening all the time and they were just on autopilot. For me, the biggest discovery was that I wasn't breathing. Despite all the feelings I could have noticed in my body, all I focused on was my intense emotional discomfort and lack of movement in my right leg.

That was a red flag. How could I not be breathing? And I was in perfect shape, so why didn't I feel my body? But I had no language, no way into the deeper messages of feeling. So don't be surprised if you feel very little and are a bit uncomfortable. Most of us want to avoid feeling; we just want to fix it not feel it.

If your response to observing your body is to dismiss it when you feel nothing, then you will continue to feel nothing. Be open minded. Give your body a chance to speak.

Jot down a few notes (on paper or digitally) about what you notice about the way you're lying on the floor today.

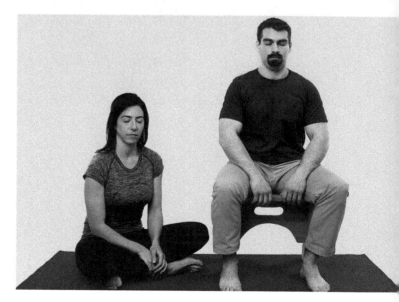

THE BODY DIALOGUE

The simple back-and-forth process between thoughts and physical feelings is what I call your Body Dialogue. In other words, it's the physical, muscular feeling of the body communicating with the vast nervous system that connects it all. We all have a Body Dialogue, and we all use it in some way every moment. Notice these thoughts; they will become valuable information.

Once we recognize our Body Dialogue, we can tweak it by giving ourselves some different directions. When you put new feelings into your body with the tools in the rest of the book, your body will begin to have choices. If we guide it, it will move away from the negative habits of pain and stress.

The Body Dialogue is happening all the time on some level, but we are not usually conscious of it. Just like your heartbeat or blinking, you don't notice it until something is wrong. You will now use this ability, as you probably have been getting feedback from your body that something needs attention. Do you notice a part of your body talking to you with discomfort, excess stiffness, or clenching? Are you holding your breath?

For example, during your Check-In you may have noticed you are holding tension in specific areas ("I seem to be clenching my right hip"). Now, as part of the Body Dialogue, you can communicate to yourself and use a cue to retrain the body with new options. Then be open to responses. It's conversational. You'll learn more about how to do this as you try out the practices in this book.

Once again, the more specific you are, the more responsive your body will be. If you say, "I am tired," even if that's true, it doesn't help your body make adjustments. We are working with a part of your brain that isn't about emotions. The Method is about retraining your body through real physical feeling, not responses to physical feelings.

I am not asking you to relax. Quite the contrary. "Relax" is more of a mental state of mind we all crave. But our physical body doesn't always respond to cues like "relax," "calm down," "be peaceful." It's hard to feel those feelings if the body is agitated in its holding positions. You can deep breathe, and that might last for a while. But why not instead notice that you are holding the muscles that will prevent you from breathing easily? Once you begin to notice that, you can breathe easily throughout your day. If you catch yourself just holding your breath, you can simply notice the muscles involved and let your body change. For now, that may sound too easy, but you will see.

Your Check-In and Body Dialogue are ways for you to acknowledge the changes in how you feel at the end of any length of time doing the Method. I encourage you to stand up and walk for a few minutes afterward and notice any parts of your body that you are engaging differently. Then add simple movements—part of the Whole Body Moves, for example, or a favorite stretch of yours—and notice if you use different muscles.

Remember, your body knows how to move. You have to get out of its way.

THE BODY FORMULA

Weight + Breath = Release of Excess Muscle Tension

Weight and breath. These are the only two cues you really need to remember to reduce excess muscle tension.

Moving the body is simply shifting your body weight in space. I use the word "weight" because we are all experiencing the resistance of gravity whether we know it or not. I don't mean "weight" like a number on the scale. I mean the feeling of the weight of the body part on the ball, or when you are sitting on a chair; the feeling of weight when standing on the floor, and the impact that has on the weight of your head going up.

During your Check-In, you may have noticed many areas of your body that don't rest on the floor. Once you notice that, you can recognize that you are fighting the laws of gravity. By creating tension in your muscles to hold yourself even when you are trying to let go, you realize the muscles aren't responding because that language—those "relax" cues—make no sense to the body.

Since it's a language to communicate with the physical body, the "cues" may seem odd. Through the Method, your brain can begin to recognize, "Oh,

I actually 'hold' myself in these positions and it's exhausting." Your body can then make the necessary adjustments. It knows how to breathe, rebalance, and move. You just need to regain some natural signals that will allow your nervous system to do this. You experience the weight of your body, and your breathing responds. This automatically begins to change the excess muscles tension and the stuck body.

Remember, you only have two options: you can resist this whole process (very common in the beginning) and hold on to the familiar stuck body, or you can allow the body to unravel some of the knots and notice how this makes you feel.

A bit about the weight. The weight is not something that we feel easily. We tend to think, "Where is the weight? Why don't I feel it?" That's why we use the ball. We go on and off the ball and cue ourselves to gradually begin to use gravity. The ball is a tool for our brain to feel a particular part of the body. As we go on and off the ball, remember gravity is something

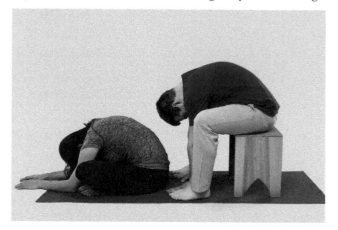

that will help us. Many people just think " Oh yes I feel that" but again don't throw these simple directions away. Linger a little longer, you may begin to get the clues that you need to unlock some of your tightest areas. But the Check-In and the Body Dialogue will help you begin.

WHAT IS TENSION?

The word "tension" comes up a lot, so I want to take some time to talk about it. Muscle tension is what we use to move the weight of the body in space. When our muscle tension is at a high level, we feel we are clenching or holding so tightly it hurts. Often in the beginning, people have no idea that they can be using a tremendous amount of muscle tension.

For me, that would be the one thing that I describe as the negative side of the body. We can take a lot of abuse. We simply get used to it. The good thing is that the body eventually does warn us with pain or nagging discomfort, so we have to change.

We need to understand that tension has a range like the volume on your phone or TV. It can be too high or too low. Each is difficult to listen to. If your tension is too high, you will find yourself unable to concentrate, distracted by the nagging discomfort, and trapped in the cycle of pain. Your breathing will be poor and your behaviors may suffer.

We sometimes think tension is bad, which makes us avoidant of using our muscles. But if your muscle tension is too low, so that there are parts of your body not involved when you move, they may be deconditioned. This can also cause discomfort in other areas.

Muscle tension is adjustable. But it must adjust; it can't get stuck. Using our muscle tension even at a high level is great, as long as we control it. We are letting ourselves move and breathe. It's when we are stuck, unable to move at one end of the scale or another because we simply are unfamiliar with the instrument, that we experience this tension getting stuck.

Most of us don't control our muscle tension very well or very consciously. It's common for us to move with as much effort to lift a small car as it is to sit at the computer. On the other hand, some of us do every movement as if we are going to fall down, with little effort. Play around with how you use your effort as you go through the book.

RECAP

Simply said:

+ The Check-In is what you feel in a given moment.

+ The Body Dialogue is the back-and-forth conversation between body and brain.

+ The Body Formula is the cues to use communicate with your body through physical sensations.

Through your senses, your body has the ability to realign. Notice how your body begins to make adjustments.

Often in exercise we address only one part of the body at a time. But the nervous system is designed so you feel your whole body at once. As you learn the Method, you may be focusing on the part of the body at hand, but still the rest of the body is with you. It sounds difficult, but think of it like reading a novel. You are reading one sentence at a time, but you still carry all the threads of the story with you throughout. This will help your body to be responsive. Remember, the responses are not arbitrary. They are specific to what you are doing and are unique to you.

By familiarizing yourself with these terms, you are getting used to the simple process of observing for a few seconds (your Check-In), noticing your thoughts (your Body Dialogue), and then finding the cues you will work with (the Body Formula). Once you get used to these terms, you will find that the body will do much of the work for you.

CHAPTER THREE

KEY AREAS

BEFORE WE MOVE on to the chapters on breathing and ball placements, let's discuss three key areas essential in relieving lower back pain: the head, the pelvis, and the rib cage.

Think of these three key areas like building blocks connected by a long flexible spine. Everything is connected. It's like putting on a Spandex jump suit. You may move your arm, but you will also feel it in your legs. There is a chain reaction throughout the body with every movement. When you become aware of this, you will notice how much easier moving is.

You may ask, "How does my head matter?" or "What does my rib cage have to do with back pain?"

Think of your nervous system like electricity.

When we have lower back pain, the key area around the pelvic muscles can feel stiff. Everything you have been learning til now is a way to "plug in" and get the current that connects all parts. If we stop the flow of movement, in turn, the stress of the movement ends up in the lower back and the knees. As with sciatic pain or herniated discs, you can feel more pressure on one side than the other.

I will point out key areas so you can use them during your ball placements, breathing, and Whole Body Moves.

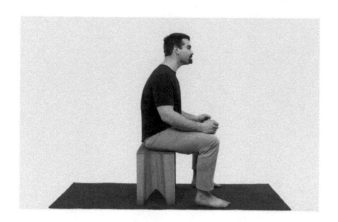

As you explore the head's connection to the rest of the body through these simple movements, be sure to initiate the movement with the head itself rather than the neck or shoulders.

1. Sit on a hard wood chair and do a Check-In.

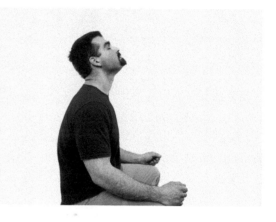

HEAD

The head is the heaviest part of the body. Most of us, due to our daily lives and habitual postures, have the head either tilted in front or in back of us. This throws off the entire length of the body and places pressure on hips, lower back, knees, and more.

The head is the line leader of your spine. Where your head goes, so goes the rest of your back. If the head is not free to find balance over what is holding it up, the entire spine is constantly straining. Then we do the back pain dance of trying to force our shoulders back or our chin up.

The head naturally wants to go up. This allows the spine to lengthen naturally.

+ Where is your head in relation to the rest of your body?

+ Do you have any sense of which muscles are involved with breathing?

2. Gradually begin to turn your head as far as you comfortably can in one direction, then return back to center. Take a moment to feel center and then turn your head to the other side.

+ How far into the rest of your body do you feel that movement?

+ Do you sense any connection to your pelvis?

3. Repeat, turning your head slowly side to side two to three times.

+ Is there a difference in the sides?

+ Do you hold your breath when moving?

Sometimes mirrors can be helpful. Many of us can't really feel the difference between initiating from one part or another. It's very common when we move to stiffen many parts of the body as we do a simple movement. Can you sense the difference between turning your head and stiffening your neck and shoulders? Gradually your body will tell you more and more as you use it with more open-mindedness to change. We are creatures of our habits. Bodies are no different.

PELVIS AND LEG JOINT

Your pelvis is the great connector between your legs and your lower back. Without loosening up this area, most people unknowingly are putting tremendous strain on their lower back.

Where most people get lower back pain is at the top of the pelvis. This is where the lumbar spine meets the top of the pelvis.

1. To start feeling how your pelvis supports your lower back, sit down and force "good posture," pushing your lower back forward.

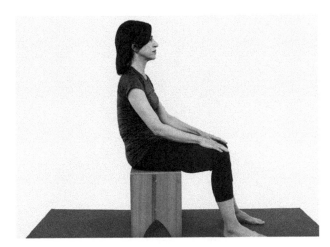

2. Many of us schlump down and back. We are unaware of the support of the pelvis.

3. Now center your body above your pelvis. This movement can help start to loosen up your pelvis and allow your body to use the pelvis to support your lower back.

The pelvis is shaped like a bowl ("pelvis" actually is the Latin word for "bowl"). Your leg joints are at the bottom of your pelvic bowl, where your legs meet your pelvis.

The foundation of all movement is your leg joint. Discovering this area of the body will give you a lifetime of relief. It also will relieve pressure on the lower back almost instantaneously once you know how to engage this area.

Most of us stand on one leg a little differently than the other. This can shorten the space between the discs, and as a result, can also activate sciatic pain. In fact, your arms and legs both will either lengthen or

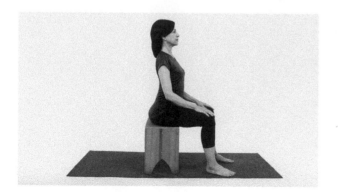

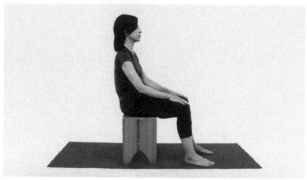

shorten the spine.

I always liken this area of the body to going down in an elevator to the basement. You may think you are on the bottom floor when then elevator stops, but then suddenly you realize there is one floor below the lobby. This is the leg joint. Most people clench without feeling the floor below the lower back—the leg joint that will take all the pressure off the lower back if you use it.

The leg joint was a big discovery for me and for most people I have worked with over the years. Clenching the muscles around the leg joint or standing on one leg more than the other can cause chronic pain in the lower back, knees, and more. But most of us don't know we are tightening this area, increasing stiffness even during exercise.

I remember watching professional dancers spend a good deal of class time just bending the knees to make this connection ruminate throughout their body. But it is not exercise alone that changes your body, but how you do the exercise and what you feel. That is why for

lower back pain, it's essential to sense this area as you use the ball placements, in sitting, doing seated body hang overs, and more.

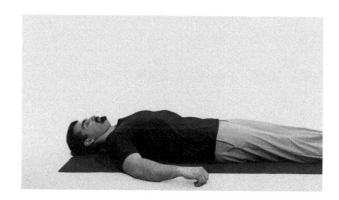

FINDING YOUR LEG JOINT WHILE LYING DOWN

1. Lie down on the floor. Start with your legs resting on the floor if possible. Notice what is on the floor and what is off the floor. Be specific. Do not force anything down.

- Notice the parts of your legs that are on the floor and those that are off the floor.

- Compare the difference under your knees.

- How much of an arch do you feel under your lower back?

- Notice where you feel your breathing.

Notice how gravity would normally have much of the body on the floor, but the knots and stiffness have shortened your muscles, preventing them from resting. We have trained ourselves to restrict our muscles with our physical habits. Even now, you can begin to stop holding so tightly by asking your body to feel the weight—not imaginary weight, but the weight of where you are bringing attention.

2. Slowly, feeling the weight of your legs, bend your knees. Did anything change?

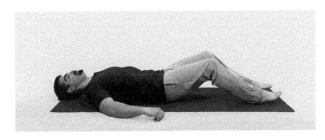

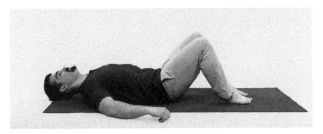

3. Stretch your legs back out. Do the spaces again change under your lower back?

4. Do this several times, each time a little more slowly, as you cue yourself to feel the weight.

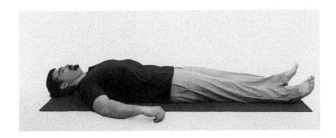

- Do your legs in some way change the muscles of your lower back (and perhaps many areas of your body)?

See if you can begin to notice how moving the legs affects many other parts of your body. This same action takes place throughout your day. The more consciously you do the movement, the more you'll discover there might be ways of doing it with less stiffness.

Helpful Hint: Try resting your hands on your hips in order to feel how the movement of the pelvis and legs change the entire body in some way.

FINDING YOUR LEG JOINT WHILE SITTING

1. Sitting on a hard wooden chair, wrap your hands around your waist. This is the top of your pelvic cavity. What you are sitting on is the bottom of your pelvis.

2. Move your knees a little closer together and then apart, keeping your feet firmly on the floor. Notice if you feel where the leg joint moves high up into the lower pelvis.

FINDING THE SITZ BONES

Most people don't realize the two bony parts at the bottom of the pelvis are where we find balance. We are always on our sitz bones, although some people roll back and some forward.

With lower back pain, most people are sitting from the top of the pelvis across the lower back. They don't feel the lower half of the pelvis, so they do a bit of a lower back dance all day. They try to lift up their body into good posture and then schlump down again because they cannot maintain it.

Throughout this book, I will continue to tell you to lift up onto the top of your sitz bones. This will take all the pressure off of the lower spine.

1. Sit on a hard chair. Notice the two bones you are resting on. Each is about the size of the tip of your index finger.

+ Can you locate both?

+ Is it painful?

2. Explore rolling behind the sitz bones and then back up.

+ Can you feel the difference between using your leg joint and lower pelvis or your lower spine?

RIB CAGE

The rib cage is right in the middle between the head and pelvis. Due to lack of breath, most people's muscles around the rib cage are like a tight ACE bandage. This makes the ribs drop like a stone on to the lower back. But no matter how much good posture you have, if you are tightly holding these muscles, somewhere in your body will suffer from lack of breath.

Most exercise programs do not encourage you to feel the difference between moving the ribs and feeling the shoulders. We will do this more for you to feel how supple this area can become and how much it will free you from sitting on your lower spine.

You will begin to lift the ribs off the lower back and create more space for herniated discs to realign and for the pressure to come off the hips and knees, which is impossible if the ribs are dropped.

We will learn in the breathing section that it's not that we have to force ourselves or lift up and then drop the body down each time we breathe. That's using the body to do the work of the diaphragmatic muscle. Your physical body will create the space. That will also take pressure off lower back, ease your day-to-day stress, and greatly improve your shape. Improved breathing also burns more calories, as it improves our metabolism.

Since excess muscle tension is at the root of all chronic pain, breathing is essential. As we relieve the excess tension and improve our breathing, our spine will lengthen. This takes the pressure off the discs and lower back. Then we will begin to move differently by using the key areas of the body.

FINDING YOUR RIB CAGE USING YOUR ARMS

1. Lie down on the floor with your arms at shoulder level.

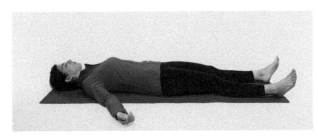

2. Slowly begin to slide your arms along the floor above your shoulder as far as you comfortably can.

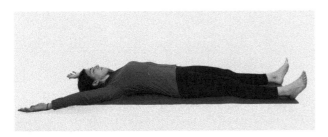

3. Gradually bring them back to where you began.

4. Then below shoulder level.

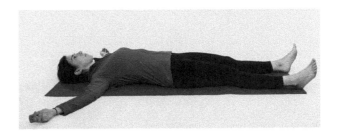

+ Did you notice your ribs move or lift?

+ Did your head arch?

Just like the leg joints connect you into your back, the shoulder joints find your back muscles when you move your arms. Feel the weight of your arms when you do this so your brain can sense the arms. If you stiffen them too much, you will disconnect from the rest of the body. The right amount of tension is not limp or locked. Experiment. You'll know it's right when your body responds easily to the movement. You will feel a chain reaction to different parts and breathing will happen naturally.

THE DIAPHRAGMATIC MUSCLE

In the middle of these three building blocks is room for your diaphragmatic muscle, the large dome-shaped muscle that attaches to the bottom of your rib cage. That muscle is usually sat on and squashed by these building blocks.

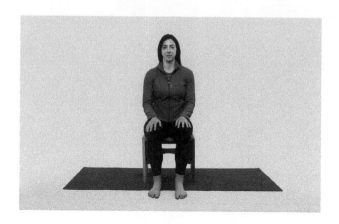

The diaphragm needs room to move freely. It can also lose tone just like any other muscle. When you begin the breathing section in chapter 4, you will begin to tone up the diaphragmatic muscle. This will begin to give you relief from the tight ACE bandage you may feel in this area. You will learn how your personal way of breathing influences your back pain.

CHAPTER FOUR

BREATHING AND YOUR BACK

BREATHING IS NOT OPTIONAL

THROUGHOUT my years of teaching, people consistently leave out the breathing piece. Even those who feel they have no problem with breathing and are experts at fitness training or yoga do not understand the relationship of breathing to relieving pain, reducing stress, and using the ability of our kinesthetic sense to constantly help us improve. We all have a lot of valuable "information" on breathing , but few have a personal experience with how their breathing is affecting them.

Before you move on to any specific routine or condition, try these breathing techniques and get a sense of how the breath changes your body. Breathing gives your body feeling, and feeling is what communicates back to your alignment system.

Since everyone breathes, most people think they are breathing. And yes, of course you are. But it is the quality of your breathing that makes movement happen and improves your mood.

If you do deep breathing and love the way it feels but then wonder why the good feelings go away, it's because your body returned to its habits. You may breathe fine when you work at it, but you can't work at it all day. I have had athletes, dancers, yoga instructors, and singers who all breathe like rock stars during their profession, but when they are done and really need the breath to be free, they go back to their habits.

Improving your understanding of your own unique way of breathing or holding your breath can greatly relieve pain, reduce muscle stiffness, improve posture, relieve stress, improve metabolism, and help you burn calories. Breathing is a way to emotionally reset and enjoy your life. It also improves the look of your body and improves your kinesthetic sense.

You do not have to make it a job to breathe more. Remember, the problem is not so much that you can't breathe as that you are preventing your body from breathing because of excess tension. You know how to breathe. Let it happen.

It is a very long list, but here are a few common things that make us hold our breath.

+ Rushing

+ Worry

+ Sitting long periods

+ Sitting at computers

+ Fears

+ Chronic pain

+ Illness

Back pain also makes us hold our breath. Pretty much any pain, illness, or anxiety makes our breathing shallow.

Stuck bodies don't breathe. In this chapter, we will begin to tone up the diaphragmatic muscle. As we talked about earlier, our bodies can be sitting right on the diaphragmatic muscle, preventing us from getting relief. Most importantly, you will notice your own unique ways you breathe (or don't breathe, like I did) by using the Check-In. These are simple observations you can do anywhere at any time.

For many of us, it's not that conscious breathing is hard to do, but it's something that is so simple we tend to overlook it. Most people want the big stuff. They want that perfect exercise. They want to have the best treatments for their back. I can tell you with certainty, if you keep an open mind and try this, you will be surprised how much relief breathing can bring.

You may begin to notice as you go through this section that your physical body begins to make adjustments as you accommodate changes to your breathing. Here is where you begin to notice the Body Dialogue. As you allow for response time from the body, the body is digesting what you are observing and the tools you are using.

BREATHING CHECK-IN

Let's check in now with your breathing. Begin by sitting or lying down. Here are a few questions to ask yourself:

+ Do you notice any muscles involved with your breathing?

+ If so, are they different on an inhalation than an exhalation?

+ Where in your body do you notice movement while you breathe? Is it more in the lower body or the shoulders?

WHAT IS OVER-BREATHING?

Many people when practicing breathing try to pull a lot of air into their body. We also do this when we are stressed. But we can "over-breathe," sucking gulps of air in and not letting it out. This actually makes the muscles tenser, and you can feel a bit lightheaded.

The *sss* sound and the *hah* sound I will describe in this section will be the exhalation. Don't worry about breathing in; you need to let your air out, and then the body will naturally pull more in. It's an easy back-and-forth process.

All of the key areas influence our breath. I'd even say that breath and posture are the same thing. And the pain we are in is reflected in our breathing.

Look at these photos of common ways people sit and stand.

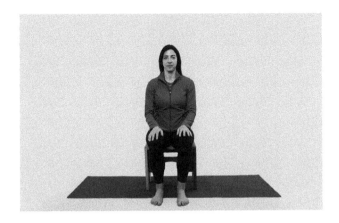

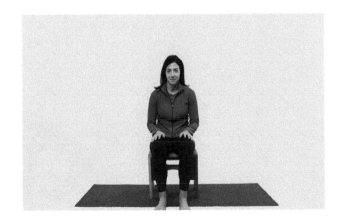

Think of the space between your ribs and pelvis as the wave a surfer rides. Notice how the ribs are crushing right into the whole breathing apparatus.

The great thing about this method is you don't look for outcomes. You do the work; the body will give you the right outcomes. Allow for the small time in between what you do and letting responses happen. No response is a response. You still give yourself that time.

When I try hard to "fix" myself, I do it all mechanically. I get no pleasure out of it, and it's a chore. But when I give up and allow myself to feel responses using the breath, the balls, the weight, and the cues, stuff happens. Whatever you feel is important. Your body may respond hours later.

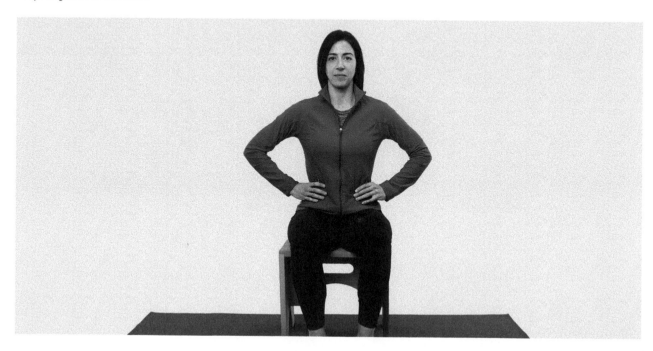

TWO EASY BREATHING TOOLS TO USE

THE *SSS* SOUND AND *HAH* SOUND

Length of time: 5-15 minutes

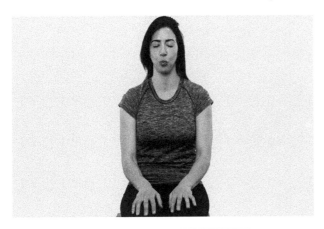

Helpful Hint: The breathing can be done anywhere. You do not have to begin sitting. You can do it lying down or sitting propped up with pillows on your bed or couch.

By making the *sss* sound, you are gradually toning the most important muscle in your body—your diaphragmatic muscle. It's important not to force these sounds or your breathing, because that sometimes reinforces the tightness in the muscles. When we strain in an attempt to get better, this actually cuts off our breathing.

Remember, you don't need to make yourself breathe in. Your body will do that naturally.

1. Check-In: Observe your breathing.

+ Do you feel where muscles are involved with breathing?

2. Begin to make a long, extended *sss* sound, like the sound of steam escaping from a tea kettle. Do this for one exhalation. Right before the end of the exhalation, stop and take notice of any responses. For example:

+ Does your breathing change in any way?

+ Do you feel it in different parts of your body?

+ Does it seem to make you yawn?

3. Make the *sss* sound again. Notice what muscles you use to make the sound. At the end of the sound, pause and give your body time to respond. If after a few breaths, there is no response, then repeat the sound.

+ Does your body begin to make any adjustments?

+ Do you need to stretch or hang forward?

4. Do a final Check-In. Notice if anything in your sitting has changed.

+ How do you know if you're doing it right? Your body will tell you. We know when something feels good or bad. If your breathing is moving more easily, you will feel better and can use that as a guide. If you are feeling worse, you may be forcing your breathing based on an old idea of what good breathing is. Keep it easygoing. If you feel good, then chances are the responses are positive. Explore that.

+ You can't mess this up. This system in the body works. It only doesn't work if you don't use it.

Helpful Hint: You don't need special clothing to practice breathing, but be aware not to have tight waistbands or jeans that might prevent you from breathing freely. Even stiff shirts or bra straps could make it difficult to let the air in.

THE *HAH* SOUND: OPEN-MOUTH BREATHING

Length of time: 5–10 minutes

1. Check-In: Begin sitting in a chair or lying down. Observe any sense of where you might notice breathing or any specifics about the way you sit when you begin.

2. Take your hand up to your open mouth and begin to make a *hah* sound, similar to fogging up a window with your own breath. Make the sound for one exhalation. Then stop, put your hand down, and notice any changes in your breathing.

3. Notice a few breaths in between to give your body a chance to respond.

4. Make the sound again. Notice the length of the sound. Notice the volume of the sound.

+ What do other muscles of your body do as you make the sound?

+ Do you tighten up your chest muscles or strain your jaw?

5. After you finish the sound, notice if your breathing changes. Do not make breathing happen, just allow the air to move in and out.

+ If you do get changes in your breathing, wait until these responses settle back to what you consider a more normal rhythm of breathing and then repeat the sound.

+ Notice if your breathing has improved.

Variation: Open-mouth breathing. When you are in bed or on the ball, you can simply ease the muscles of your jawbone and let the weight of your jaw open your mouth. Exhale.

SOME COMMON RESPONSES TO DOING THE BREATH WORK

+ Your eyes might water.

+ You may want to stretch.

+ Some people get lightheaded.

+ You may notice the muscles along your back getting cranky until the breath moves in.

As you continue to go through the book, pick and choose what will work best for you based on the pain you're experiencing now.

RECAP

+ Forcing deep breathing is not necessary.

+ Breathing is a way to feel your stuck body and reverse the cycle of pain.

+ You can do it anywhere.

Many of us hold our breath. We do this for reasons of stress, pain, and postural habits. When we hold our breath, the diaphragmatic muscle is minimally moving and the muscles along the spine begin to shorten. This causes the discomfort in many areas of our lower back and lower body.

PART

2

Up to now I hope you are finding the easy back-and-forth process with the breathing. The same process applies to the next two chapters. In Part 2 You will be incorporating breathing with Whole Body Moves and Ball placements. When doing the ball placements, you will also get more familiar with the key areas as you move ahead and the directions. For example, you will have an initial Check-In for you to compare with at the end of your time on the ball. Feel the weight and allow for responses. Acknowledging specific changes, as small as you may think they are, trains your brain–body connection to move differently throughout your day.

When on the ball, notice your thoughts. They are communicating to your physical body and will be a way for you to use the Body dialogue. If you notice you stop breathing and are thinking about the rest of your day, bring yourself back. Use your cues from the Body Formula. If your thoughts are reactive and negative, your body will not feel directed or sense you are allowing it to make changes.

Linger longer, take your time to continue to improve the kinesthetic sense. There is no benefit to trying to fix and force. Giving yourself time allows your body to make adjustments.

Think of your cell phone connecting to service. Sometimes you move a little here or there and it sounds totally different. Your body may move a bit and shift on the ball. Remember, your body knows how to "undo" what we do to it. Let it have its say.

When things don't feel right, respond to that as well. Try a different ball placement. Just like in any dialogue, sometimes one person speaks and the other person listens. It's not a monologue where you just tell your body what to do.

Let's begin now with what some of my students have described as "stretching without stretching." I call these Whole Body Moves. This is a reminder that when you exercise, or move in any way, you want to retrain yourself to feel or let the entire body get involved.

WHOLE BODY MOVES

As you sense more parts of your body, you begin to take the pressure off the lower back. Lower back muscles are extremely strong sturdy muscles but they can't do the work for the whole body. This is actually the way your body is designed to move. Focusing on one part may work for directional reasons, but whatever you are doing, the whole body is either helping your or hindering you from moving freely. The nervous system works as a whole interconnected unit. Think of someone playing a song, there are hundreds if not thousands of notes. If they had to stop on each note you would not hear the melody. Your body moves in a similar way. When you use the Whole Body Moves you will feel the shifts of weight, notice key areas, and have time to allow breathing to move throughout your body naturally. You begin to trust that your brain can do a similar process a musician does with playing an instrument. You move freely using all the different feelings and directions you have learned. You will lengthen your muscles, not lock them. You will reach and not be rigid.

It sounds more complicated, but as you do the Method you will find it happens very naturally, as you use gravity and allow your breathing to respond naturally. For purposes of pain, when you allow gravity to work with the weight of your body you will bend deeper in the joints. This allows the spine to lengthen not lock and hold. You will begin to feel key areas that make standing and sitting easier. It will become clear when you are straining because you are not feeling the weight and breathing.

Chapter 6 will introduce you to eight basic ball placements. Notice how the balls along with breathing and the cues bring to life the key areas of your body. Let the part of your body on the ball feel supported. Some areas of your body may feel as if you have been squeezing a tennis ball very hard in your fist for many years. As you rest the weight on the ball, you are gradually allowing your muscles to loosen their grip. Begin to notice the easing of your tightest muscles. Oddly enough, some of our tightest areas feel the least. They are part of our habits and we don't notice what we are doing until the pain, the warning signal begins to give valuable information.

Because lying on the floor seems easier than sitting, and we are not required to do much, many of us think just by lying down we already have no more stuck body. The floor is easier, because our habits are not working so hard to keep us standing or sitting. But all of the excess muscle tension is still there.

This is a great opportunity to notice how and where you hold tightly and let some of those clenched muscles readjust and take pressure off the lower back. The sciatic nerve is greatly affected by the clenching and stiffness in the muscles. The more you squeeze the muscles, the more contracted the spaces will be between the vertebrae. This will exacerbate sciatic pain and herniated discs. You may begin to feel that the knees and hips are different on each side. Compare the differences. Small changes can create huge improvement, because you are not simply working the surface muscles but the way they hold your skeleton in place. Gradually you go into deeper layers of muscles that affect the skeletal alignment.

Enjoy this section. If one Whole Body Move or Ball placement doesn't feel right to you, move on to another.

TYPES OF LOWER BACK PAIN

Here are three different kinds of lower back pain you might be experiencing. This will help you choose what is best for you at this time. You will see the stars next to the ball placements to correspond to the level of difficulty you are in need of at this time.

+ Acute lower back pain is after you recently hurt your back. You may not be able to get on the balls until the back gradually begins to heal. Acute pain takes a certain amount of time to heal. You may need medical attention and recommendations for care. Do not force yourself to stretch and do not go on the balls. Gentle breathing is always effective. One star is the most gentle, but even that may not be recommended until you feel ready.

+ Chronic lower back pain is when, after several months, you still have pain. You can begin to get differing options on what to do. You find you have modified your lifestyle to accommodate the pain. Because pain is very subjective, it's not always easy for doctors to know what we're experiencing. This is where you need to begin to understand how you yourself experience pain.

+ Occasional lower back pain comes and goes. Your back can feel like it is always stiff, always uncomfortable. Or you might be accommodating your day-to-day activities because of worries the back pain you had at one time will return. You might find certain activities bring it on like gardening or sports training.

When using this book, please be aware that the Method is very gentle, but certain ball placements may accommodate you more than others. The stars are a suggestion. DO not feel because there is one star that it won't be beneficial, or that three stars are better for you. Understanding the method is how it will benefit you, whether one star or three. These are to inform you that there can be extremely tight areas of the body that there is no reason to force changes.

* Very easy to do , a great way to begin to understand how to do the method

* * Challenging to more areas of the body: you understand the method and are ready to rest the ball under more areas of the body without holding your breath or stiffening.

* * * Requires more understanding of the Method

CHAPTER FIVE

WHOLE BODY MOVES

REACHING, bending, squatting, and twisting are movements that use the entire interconnected system of muscles, bones, and nerves. Think of the muscles over your bones like wearing a whole-body sweater that stretches. Each time you reach your arm, you can feel it into your waist or hips. Your muscles want to do the same thing. Did you ever bend over and a tight belt prevented you from moving, or a tight necktie made it hard to turn your head? A similar process is happening with the body where our habits prevent us from moving.

Whole Body Moves incorporate key areas of the body that can be gridlocked like cars at an intersection in a traffic jam. The cues of breathing and weight will help you notice the feeling of the gridlock, and the balls will help you unlock that direction.

Whole Body Moves are a reminder that the body doesn't separate into parts, but that every movement is a whole body movement. Think of your vertebrae like links in a chain. They are all connected and as one moves others respond as well unless your chain gets stuck. Whole body moves are designed for you to feel the "stuck" areas of the body and allow gravity and breathing to gradually stretch them where they can then "link" back into the rest of the body.

Because most of us have strong habits of movement, we will need to use the Body Dialogue to cue ourselves: "Oh, there's a joint there" or "I can actually lengthen and not lock my muscles." Words have a great impact on the body.

In this chapter, we are going to focus on a few Whole Body Moves. It's not so much the movement that you care about as the feelings that you get when doing them. Those are your body's responses. It's the same back-and-forth we had during the breathing chapter. It's like getting a frequency on the radio— you dial it in a little here, a little there. There are moments when your body might respond abruptly, "This is wrong; it hurts." That is not your body telling you "Never do this movement again"—it's your body telling you do the movement differently. Remind yourself to breathe, to feel the weight. These little cues enable the body to be responsive. You don't need to do anything more than use the cues and let yourself respond.

Many of us get tighter when we "try" to force a stretch, which actually reinforces the stuck body. Using the Whole Body Moves and the breathing techniques begins to give you a sense of how easily the body can move when you use gravity. You will be ready to get on the ball in chapter 6!

How do you know if you are doing it right? You will not need to hold your breath and it will not hurt— although moving parts of your body differently can give you a feeling of discomfort.

When you begin to bend at the leg joint, your hamstrings will stretch. If not, all the pressure is in the lower spine. For example, many of us are shocked at how stiff the hamstrings are when the hamstrings begin to stretch using the Whole Body Moves. It can seem scary. Go at it slowly. Your leg joints will probably make you aware of how tight your hamstrings are. As you gradually lengthen these, they will support and begin a lifetime of relief.

You will use the specific cues from the Body Formula, like feeling the weight of the part that's bending. Sense how you do it, and notice if you are forcing or straining. Gradually, you will find the "feeling" in the legs. They won't be locked or stiff. They will support you. As you get more and more response from these Whole Body Moves, your lower back pain will drift farther and farther away.

When you have chronic pain, you sometimes limit the movements you do because you worry that if they hurt, something is wrong with the movement. Unfortunately, that paints us into a corner and we move less and less. Moving less and less means your body will complain more and more. Stop and observe when you feel discomfort. Notice whether you like to hold your breath during a Whole Body Movement, or if you like to fight gravity and "hold" certain parts very tightly. If you can feel gravity helping you, then your breathing will bring necessary circulation into those tense muscles. Discomfort can be a direction. Part of learning anything is experimenting. By gradually using all different parts of the Method, the breathing, Whole Body Moves, and the balls, you begin to have options. The discomfort may be from forcing, a part of a familiar way many of us move. When you stop and use some of the new feelings or physical experiences you have had, you might be surprised that the discomfort eases and improves.

I have watched thousands of people and also have experienced this process myself. Remember that the thoughts are part of pain. I had to be very clear with myself, because I was always ready to drive myself to the emergency room with every sensation. With this Method, you can gradually build confidence. See if you have thoughts that you are hurting yourself, that your pain is never going away, and if you do the wrong movement you will be in chronic pain for longer periods of time. Ask yourself if those thoughts are helping you or even logical.

When I teach, I ask people to speak up and share what they feel. I remind them that their feelings may be inaccurate. Checking in and being open to the process allows us to realize we have to let the body work. Let's start with seated body hang over and finding our sitz bones for relief. The seated body hang over gives you a sense of using the deep connection the leg joint creates throughout the body.

Sitting is a good place to start. Because we sit a lot during the day, you can use this Whole Body Move to reset your body even when you're not in the middle of a session. When done using the messages of the Body Formula, a seated body hang over connects you deeply to the muscles throughout the body. It uses the weight of your body and your breath.

Remember, there are three parts to relieving chronic lower back pain. Notice your thoughts, your breathing, and your physical body. We want to break it down so it's clear what seems to be influencing how you move. Your thoughts, your muscles, your breathing.

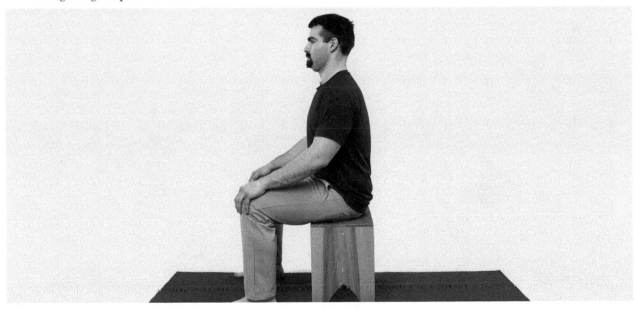

SEATED BODY HANG OVER

Key Area: Pelvis and Leg Joint

1   Check-In: Sitting at the edge of a hard chair, notice your breathing. Rest your hands on your upper leg joints to get a sense of where you will bend from.

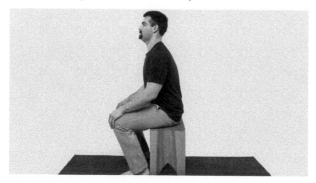

2   Bend forward. Let gravity do its job. Think of folding; let your arms hang gradually. You can hang over for as long as you are at ease; longer is not necessary. Notice the way you do it. Another option is to reach one arm and then the other to stretch the whole body.

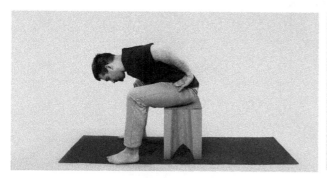

3   Gradually bring your whole body up. Lift the pelvis and allow the head to come up as well.

+   Remember the key area of the pelvis and leg joints? Do you lift from there or from your neck or lower back?

4   Take a minute to notice how you balance on your sitz bones. Is there anything different? Feel free to take a few minutes to make the *sss* sound. Remember, your breathing is a big part of how easily your body will move. It's not hard, but it is different to not hold the breath.

+   Repeat two more times and use the cues, feeling the weight of your body give in to gravity, letting your leg joint bend.

+   Notice if you bend deeper in the leg joint and lengthen more of your body each time you come up. Feel yourself lifting, perching on the tip of your sitz bones. Allow your head to float up and sense your breathing.

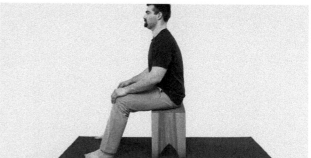

TROUBLESHOOTING: OBSERVE YOUR KNEES IN RELATION TO YOUR FEET.

+ Open the thighs so the knees are over the second or third toes.

+ If you don't feel your leg joint, or cannot open your knees over your toes, your feet may be too far apart.

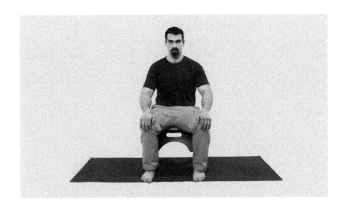

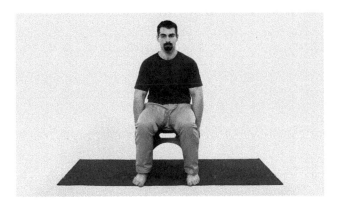

TROUBLESHOOTING: FIND THE CONNECTION OF THE LEG JOINT TO THE PELVIS.

+ Begin sitting on a bench or hard wood chair. (see photos) Notice where your feet are in relation to your knees. Leg muscles can be very tight and lock the pelvis in a position putting strain on the lower spine. Place the knees so if you dropped a plum line from the tip of your knee downward, it would point over your second or third toes.

+ If your feet are too far apart it may be hard to do this. Have your feet hip joint distance apart. Then slowly move your knees towards each other and away about the width of your foot. See if you feel movement in your pelvis. This is where you bend from. This is far from where most of us bend, putting strain on the lower back. This will take some time to find, but once you find it you never lose it. These muscles gradually give as you use the cues, direct your body to feel the weight and let yourself breathe.

+ It is much easier to do seated than standing. Once the knee is aligned over the toes, then do your seated body hangover. Using gravity along with the weight of your body will lengthen the lower spine.

REACHING ARMS

Key Area: Rib Cage

Lengthening the spine with Whole Body Moves while breathing is excellent for also lengthening the muscles along the spine and taking pressure off the lower back.

your posture, relieves much upper body stiffness and improves breathing.

Any movement with your arms is going to affect how your spine moves. This Whole Body Move gives

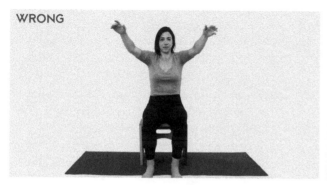

WRONG

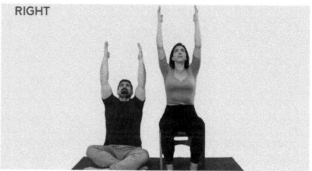

RIGHT

In the right photo there is no need to use the shoulders to lift the arms. The person allows the arms to connect to the back and it will lift the spine. This takes pressure off of the lower back.

In the left photo you will notice what is more common.

More common is to lift the shoulders instead of connecting to the back. The shoulders then get tighter and tighter.

Use a mirror when you do this to see which picture is more like you. Repeating the whole body move, using your kinesthetic sense to feel more parts of the body will allow the body to break that habit. It also enhances

you that direct sense of how connected you are to your back. It also gives you better balance and posture as well as being a great way to relieve stress.

When you begin this movement, bring your attention not only to your arms. Your arms have no ability to lift without the rest of your body and your breathing. Your body knows that and cannot respond in a positive way if you are isolating one part. That way of doing things is in the past.

And let's change the dialogue as we go through this. Use words like "stretch," not "strain," "lengthen," not "lock."

1   Sit on the floor or on a chair or bench. Make the *sss* sound before you start. Begin a brief Check-In. Notice where you feel your breathing.

2   Begin to notice the feeling of your arms hanging along your sides. Feel free to use your hands to guide you as you did in seated body handover. Perhaps put them side by side.

3   Gradually, while feeling the weight of your arms, reach your hands to the ceiling. Notice how you do the movement. Only go as far as you comfortably can. Then gradually let the weight of your arms ease back down alongside your body.

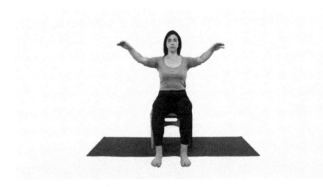

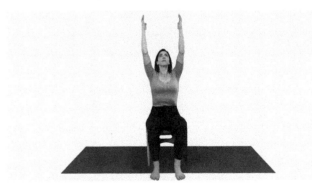

+   Do you stiffen your neck?

+   Do you begin the movement with the shoulders?

4   Try this three or four times. Explore, experiment, use the way you move, and notice if you are repeating movements the same way or incorporating some of the new feelings from the Method. The first time you do this is normally your habit of movement.

+   Did you hold your breath?

+   Did you notice any response with other parts of your body?

+   Were you straining or forcing the arms or shoulders to go higher?

+   Do your arms rest closer to your sides?

+   Has your breathing changed?

Helpful Hint: Use a mirror to see how you do the movement. The moment you begin your movement, notice what happens to other parts of your body. You can change where you bring your attention. If your thoughts are all about forcing, fixing, holding, or straining, change these cues to ones like weight, balance, lengthening, and reaching.

As with all movements in the Method, give yourself a chance to let the body respond before you repeat.

Modification: Bring the arms to shoulder level only. Before you begin again, feel free to make the *sss* sound. If you felt you were forcing or straining, only go to shoulder level the next time you try. When your arms get to shoulder level, give a little reach and then gradually let them back down.

Helpful Hint: When you return your arms to your side, you do not need to compress the key area of your waistline.

Remember, what is different with the Miracle Ball Method is you gain more by noticing how you do things than by forcing yourself to change. Just like most things in life, when you see the problem clearly, it's easy to change.

For example, a simple movement like reaching the arms might hurt your shoulders, so you tighten your shoulders more. You then have thoughts that might be directing you to give up and further hold your breath. That is the cycle most people live in. But with some different directions, you will have a completely different response.

Now whether you are golfing or walking, learn to bring your attention to the feeling of all the parts, especially key areas and your breathing. This is the way your body works best. When you do it differently, you will begin to feel clarity that what you did made the change and took the pressure off the lower back. Then you can find ways to reinforce movements that you do differently and create long-term change.

STANDING BODY HANG OVER

Key Area: Leg Joints and Hamstrings

Do this practice two to three times a day. Make sure you have a secure floor and footwear so as not to slide. It may take a few months before your body gradually learns it can get more relief by not fighting the weight of the body bending at the leg joint.

Do not hold your breath.

1   Have your legs a little farther than hip joint distance apart. While standing, take a moment to check in.

2   With your feet planted firmly on the ground and leg muscles working, gradually let your body bend forward. Begin to feel all the key areas of your body until you fold at your leg joint. Hang for just a brief time.

3   Gradually bring your body back up to standing. Notice how you do this. Do you begin with your shoulders? Your low back? Are you holding your breath? Once you come up to standing, take notice of how you stand. Listen to any adjustments your body wants to make.

4   Repeat and use gravity. Can you let the weight of your body, and your experience of where your leg joints are, help you to bend deeper in the hip, allowing pressure off the lower back? If your lower back is doing all the work, come back up and try it again, putting your hands on your hips.

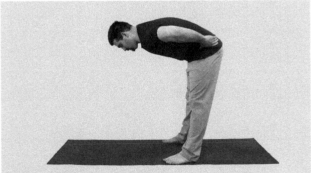

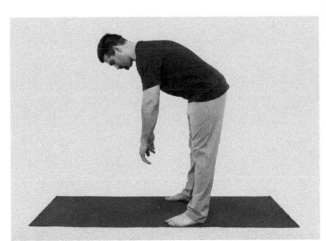

5   On the final time you come back up, lift your pelvis up onto the legs. Take a walk around the room and notice if you move or breathe differently. Repeat two more times and use the cues, feeling the weight of your body give in to gravity, letting your leg joint bend.

TROUBLESHOOTING: STRAIGHTEN THE LEGS WITHOUT LOCKING THE KNEES

Most people do not want to straighten their legs because someone told them not to or because they are too stiff. Straightening the legs is different than stiffening. Stiffness is not strength. By accommodating bent knees, we actually lose the support for our lower back. Learning how to straighten the legs will be easier after being on the balls and breathing because the muscles will begin to get more supple

You can practice the standing hangover two ways, with knees lifted and legs straight or with bent knees. DO not force them to straighten by stiffening and locking the knees. See if you can lift the thigh muscles, incorporate the feeling of the leg joint and you're breathing. How your feet anchor you is also part of this movement. This is important because the legs have a strong connection to supporting your lower back. Too many of us are told, just let your knees bend. I understand that because no one wants you to force something and hurt yourself. But that also reinforces weakness in the legs which will not help your lower back long term. This is a gradual process that you will get better at.

Remember all movement is a whole body move-ment. Use this challenge to discover how you have trained yourself to move a certain way and begin to explore by using some of the parts of the body you have noticed on the balls and while breathing.

But straightening the legs is important to have a sense that your legs are supporting you. Without this feeling, the lower back will complain and get tighter and tighter through your lifetime.

Here are some ways for you to feel you are using your legs and not stiffening them.

+ Do not lock your knees. Instead, feel they are lifting with your thigh muscles.

+ Use the feeling of your feet on the floor for an oppositional stretch.

+ Do not think "go limp" as many people do; your legs are your support.

+ Cue yourself to feel that you are exploring bending at the leg joint. Your brain will begin to find that part. Make sure your knees are not rolling in or out.

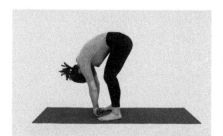 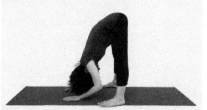 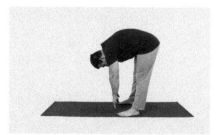

WHOLE BODY TWIST

Key Area: Rib Cage

This Whole Body Move loosens up the tight ACE bandage most of us feel wrapped around our torso. You will learn to let gravity help you as you feel the weight of the middle of the body roll back slightly, opening up the chest to the ceiling. This is an excellent way to find the middle of the body. Follow the directions. Do not force the shoulder to do the work of the rib cage.

   You will probably find you are extremely tight. Don't stay long in a place that feels forced. Get a slower start; notice how the parts connect. Spend about five to ten minutes with this Whole Body Move.

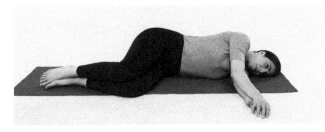

1   Check-In: Begin lying on the floor or in bed. Make the *sss* sound and check in. Acknowledge what parts of your body are resting on the floor and what areas you might be straining to hold off the floor. Be specific.

   +   Notice where you touch the floor and where your body is off the floor.

   +   Notice your breathing.

2   Roll onto your right side. If you are in pain on the right side, begin on the left side. Many roll on top of the bottom shoulder, causing more pain. Hold your body slightly back from being on top of the shoulder.

   +   Much of how we hold our posture during the day is very clear lying on our side. You can use this as a way to improve your posture. Lie there for a moment. What do you notice?

3   Gradually reach your left hand forward, on top of right hand. Begin to trace a half-circle along the floor over your head.

4   Gradually begin to move your arm behind your head as your ribs and upper body softly twists; do not force. Only go as far as you comfortably can, and then return.

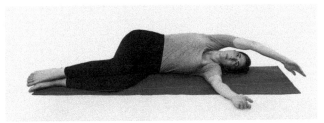

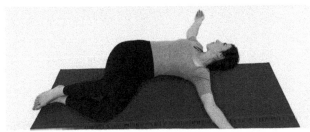

5   At the top of the circle, see if you can begin to take your arm behind your head (still about an inch off the floor). What happens?

6   Begin to gradually bring your arm back to your side. Notice your breathing and how your whole body moves. Rest for a minute and let the body adjust.

Modification: Feel free to put a rolled-up towel or blanket under the side of your head, but just high enough to be comfortable.

Troubleshooting: A crucial mistake most adults make is to try to force the movement with their shoulder rather than letting the connecting of their arms move into the back. Remember your whole body moves your arms. Most people try to force their whole body to move with the shoulders. Try it again, letting the head roll, the rib cage roll, then return back.

Repeat three times on each side.

+   The first time, sense your way of moving, your habit.

+   The second time, change the focus and the use the cues.

+   The third time, again use the cues, let yourself breathe in between, and don't work so hard (it's not helping).

Many of the Whole Body Moves reveal the ways we are stuck. Lying on your side may reflect how you hold yourself all day long even when walking or standing. Is your head forward or back? Are you curled in a ball? Is the bottom shoulder stiff or sore? Imagine a mirror on the ceiling. Can you describe your shape? Lengthen out a bit by using something under your head to lengthen your neck.

See if you can use the cues to dialogue differently with your body. If you don't begin to change the dialogue with your body using different directions, you will not improve. It may seem awkward at first, but you have been unknowingly training yourself for years. Don't be negative if you feel your stuck body. That is great! You cannot move what you ultimately do not feel.

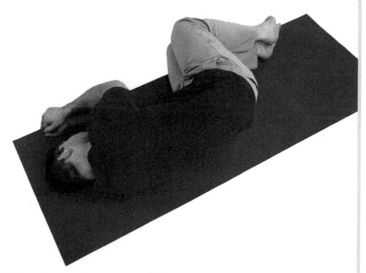

HEAD HANGING FORWARD

Key Area: Head

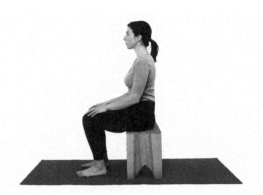

This Whole Body Move takes pressure off of many areas of the body. You will discover that lifting the head lengthens the whole body. Most of us lift the head by shortening the neck and stiffening the shoulders. It's part of holding the breath, and it's a familiar posture for those who sit for long periods.

The Whole Body is beautifully designed to support the head. The secret of doing this movement is really allowing yourself to feel the head. Use your cues. Ask your brain to feel the weight of the head. Otherwise, you'll repeat your habit of movement.

Once you use the weight of the head to connect to the rest of your body, you will find you can allow it to float up and lengthen the spine naturally. This allows the other key areas to make adjustments. There is no longer pressure on the lower back.

1   Check-In: Begin sitting in a chair or cross-legged on the floor. Check in with your sitting. Remember, don't force your posture; simply notice.

+   Notice how you balance your head in relation to the rest of your body.

+   Do you notice any muscles involved with breathing?

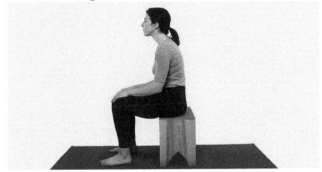

2   Gradually begin to let the weight of your head bend forward.

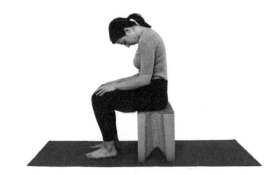

3   Stay there for a moment or two, and then gradually bring your head back up. Gradually raise head.

+   Notice how other parts of your body responded. Are you in the same place?

+   Did you stop breathing?

4   Allow the weight of your head to bend forward again.

+   Is it heavier?

+   Are more parts of your body involved?

+   Take five to ten minutes and repeat this four or five times. Give yourself time to notice other key areas.

+   Do the neck muscles stretch?

+   When you lift the head up, does it lengthen other parts of your body? On the final time you come back up, lift your pelvis up onto the legs. Take a walk around the room and notice if you move or breathe differently. Repeat two more times and use the cues, feeling the weight of your body give in to gravity, letting your leg joint bend.

TROUBLESHOOTING: USE YOUR WHOLE BODY TO LIFT YOUR HEAD.

Many of us use the neck alone to lift the head. Notice the two pictures.

Place your hand on the top of your head when upright. (You can even use a book or a plate.) Try to lengthen through your body to reach your hand. Sense the chain reaction to the movement of your head. Remove your hand and let the neck muscles respond. Notice if any part of your body feels different. Do your ribs move back as the head goes forward?

Many of us think of alignment as being stiff, like holding a particular posture or position. But it is better to have a thousand "wrong" movements than simply being stuck in a posture or position. The body is extremely forgiving when you move. It makes thousands of adjustments all day long unless you are stuck in place. Your body will work it out as you find more parts of your body and use them. You can do any of the Whole Body Movements throughout your day. Anytime you feel you are returning to the stuck place, spontaneously allow your body to move. At first, it might seem rehearsed and awkward. Soon enough, the body will find it refreshing, the pain will lessen, your shape will improve, and you will get reenergized in the middle of your day

LEG TO SIDE

All Key Areas

This move is excellent for lower back pain as well as gaining a feeling of lengthening your sides. Many of us can experience two very different sides. This can be in the legs primarily, but the waist and the shoulders are also involved.

1   Lie on your back with your arms out at shoulder level.

2   Bend your knees, with your feet hip distance apart.

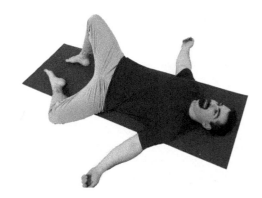

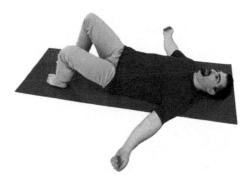

3   Begin to feel the weight of your left thigh open out to the left. Gradually allow it to rest on the floor.

4   The other leg must stay in position along with your feet. You may let the right foot lean to the outside. But do not allow the feet to go limp. This will detach the connection throughout the body.

5   Gradually return the leg to where it began. Notice your breathing. Allow the rest of your body to respond. Repeat slowly several times.

+   Do you notice changes throughout your back and up your sides?

+   Think "lengthen," not "lock," and notice the key areas of your leg joints changing on each side as your pelvis must move to allow the leg to stretch.

6   Stretch your legs out and compare sides. Make the *sss* sound. What do you notice? Repeat on the other side.

TENSION EXTENSION

All Key Areas

Gain strength in new areas of the body to take with you when you return to your daily activities. After any of your Whole Body Moves on the floor or any ball placements, try this.

1   Gradually reach your arms and legs in opposite directions. Reach away from the core or middle of your body. Think of lying in the middle of a circle. Reach your hands and feet towards the edges of the circle. The lengthening from one end to the other creates much needed length along the muscles of the spine and gives your low back relief.

   +   Begin with the right side, slowly reaching the right hand and foot at the same time. Then alternate to the left.

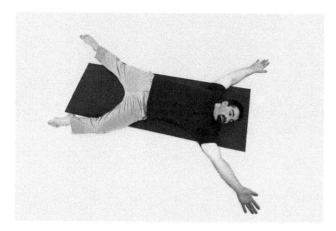

2   Feel the chain reaction throughout your body.

3   If you tend to strain one part, stop and reassess. Repeat it differently

We are learning about tension here. You can strain and stiffen, or you can lengthen your muscles in a direction. By doing this Whole Body Move, you move the middle of your body and you'll gain much relief in the lower back. This area needs to feel it has the ability to move. If you sit on it, compress it, or unknowingly shorten it, you will feel the effects in your lower back, hips, knees, and many other parts of your body.

You must have equal effort to feel it in the middle. Many of us use a tremendous amount of effort in either the upper body or the lower body. Some of us will strain our shoulders to try to get a stretch. Think of tying your shoelaces. You learned years ago that you give equal effort to get the bow in the middle. This applies to the body as well. Match the weaker area. If your legs and feet tend to work less, then match that effort with the shoulders. Do not try to strain both ends of the body.

CHAPTER SIX

BALL PLACEMENTS

THE ball placements bring everything together. Because the nervous system is that electricity connecting all parts of your body, the ball is the conduit for you to feel all the key areas. It's like being on a car ride, and you are taking it all in.

The ball does not have to go where your lower back hurts in order to improve how you feel. In fact, that might be the wrong place to put the ball. If you have pain on the ball, you will activate the cycle of pain. You will not be able to let the weight of your body rest.

Before doing any ball placements, start with your Check-In and notice your breathing.

You do not have to go through every ball placement. Find the ones that help you to feel your stuck body and the ones that allow you to enjoy your body's ability to feel and allow your body to move freely after. Incorporate your breathing throughout.

Explore the three key areas, use your cues, and end with a Whole Body Move if possible. Less is definitely more. We are trained to think that if we don't force or fix, then we are weak. You are not going easy in order to be soft on yourself but to allow this miraculous ability your body has to retrain you to enjoy moving.

It's as simple as listening to a great song. No matter how many times you listen, it still gives you feeling. Each time, you hear things you didn't the time before. Your body is the same way. But if you begin to overanalyze, the body will not have the experience, just as if you began to overanalyze the song, you might not enjoy it.

One of my students recently said the truest thing

and didn't even know it. She said, "I never knew I clench the muscles on my entire right side." She looked so sad. Although she wanted nothing more than to have her pain gone, she said, "I can't even imagine living without it." Change is challenging for most of us. It's not challenging physically as much as emotionally. We get stuck in the pain, the thoughts, and the way we live our lives as a result of our pain. We are complicated beings. Go easy. You will be fine. But you will learn a lot about yourself too.

You can order the balls at www.miracleballmethod.com, see videos on different placements, and read testimonials from doctors and other students who have loved the Method.

In every ball placement, remember these cues:

+ Notice the weight of the part of your body resting on the ball.

+ Let it get heavier, feel the weight of this part of your body.

+ Notice if your body makes any small movements as you allow the muscles to be supported by the ball. I call this a gradual "unraveling" of the tight muscles along the lower back.

+ Do you feel any response in other parts of your body?

+ Have you decided to hold your breath?

+ Where do you feel breathing?

Before or after any of the ball placements, you have the option to begin sitting and do a Check-In. This could be thirty seconds or you could take a few minutes to make the *sss* sound and notice your breathing.

A Check-In is also very useful when you are done with any time on the balls. Discerning differences even after short periods of time is what allows you to carry the changes with you during your day. More parts of your body get involved with moving, and the habits begin to be replaced with freedom to move.

BACK ON THE BALL OPTION 1

Key Area: Pelvis and Leg Joint   Star rating: *****

1   Check-In: Lie down on the floor and check in. You may want to make the *sss* sound.

2   Gradually bend your knees and rest your feet on the floor.

3   Slowly roll your pelvis to the side and place a ball in the middle back of your pelvis. (You can use two balls if using one causes pain.)

+   Stay on the ball for a short period of time, about one minute depending on your responses.

+   Make the *sss* sound. Notice if you feel any sinking of your lower back. Would you describe your body from the ball to your shoulders as arched like a bow, a flat line, or sinking like a hammock?

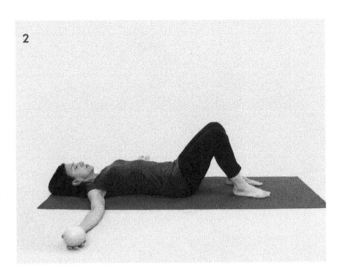

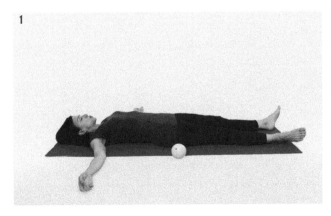

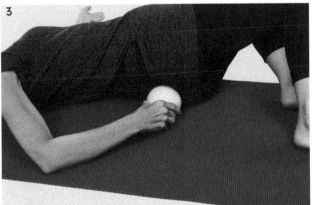

4   Gradually begin to arch at your beltline, allowing your pelvis to roll down toward the floor. Then let gravity return it to where your body feels the weight more.

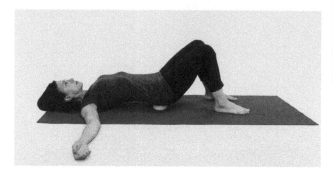

+ Does each side feel different when you do this?

+ Do you feel anything in the other key areas, your head and your rib cage?

+ Where do you feel breathing?

5   Roll your pelvis over to the side. Quickly remove the ball and stretch your legs out. Notice how you rest on the floor now.

+ Has your breathing changed?

+ Can you let your legs rest more easily on the floor?

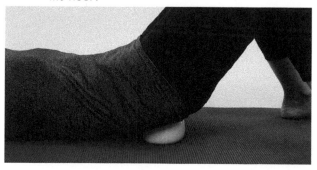

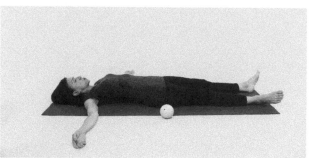

+ Compare the feelings with what you noticed when you did your initial Check-In.

The leg joint is the great connector between lengthening and realigning the lower back muscles on each side.

6   Repeat this ball placement, adding a slight rolling of the pelvis back and forward. Take your time in order to use new muscles to lengthen your back.

This movement is similar to rolling behind and in front of your sitz bones (page 36). You do not have to clench or lift off the ball, but more feel the shift of the pelvis. Then leave the ball there and slide your legs out in front of you.

Sciatica: For those with sciatic pain, notice if you feel a difference in the leg joint when doing the movement on the ball on each side. Does the side with the sciatica feel different? Does your pelvis lean into that side or the other? Notice your rib cage. The next time you do the small movements, sense if you can move the sides more evenly based on your responses.

BACK ON THE BALL OPTION 2

Key Area: Pelvis and Leg Joint   Star rating: ★ ★

A definite feeling takes place through the whole body during this ball placement.

Repeat getting on the ball as in option 1, steps 1–3.

1   Lift your feet off the floor and bend at the leg joint. Feel the weight of the pelvis on the ball. Make the *sss* sound.

2   Allow the weight of your thighs to open if you feel anchored on the ball. Then return your legs back together. Repeat this three times. Use the entire leg, not simply your knees.

3   Take your feet down one at a time.

4   Stretch your legs out and notice your breathing. Make the *sss* sound.

   +   If you are comfortable, you can leave the ball there. When you are ready, slowly roll to the side and quickly remove the ball.

5   Notice any changes when resting on the floor now

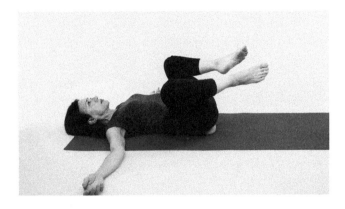

This placement requires more of a shift of weight. The weight of your legs dramatically stretches the lower back muscles. Avoid the feeling of holding; instead, think "bending" and "breathing."

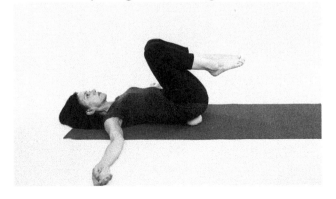

Especially when opening the legs, there should be no pain in the knees. If there is, you are directing yourself to open the hip with the knee. Try again and allow the inner thigh muscles to open the leg. Developing these muscles is essential to lengthening the clenched and shortened muscles that many experience on one side. This can put strain all the way down one side of the body, affecting the knees, hips, and lower back. As you repeat opening the thighs and then bringing the legs back together, explore moving them with equal effort, regaining a balance and changing your habit

BACK ON THE BALL OPTION 3

Key Area: Pelvis and Leg Joint; Rib Cage   *Star rating:* **★ ★ ★**

This is a challenging placement, because the body will be moving to slide over the ball or balls. (Be aware that they can get tied up in loose T-shirts.) Then you will be resting the balls under key areas like the rib cage, which can be the tightest muscles of our body. Do not feel this is something you should do right away until you feel comfortable with your breath and knowing how to give in to the weight. Remove the balls at any time if it gets to be too much. Some people love this.

1   Repeat getting on the ball as in option 1, steps 1–3.

2   Rest with your feet on the floor and breathe.

3   Gradually, using your own body weight, slide the ball up the back just an inch or two. Rest.

4   Continue gradually along the entire back of your body. Then remove the ball.

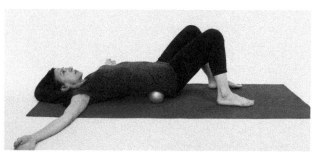
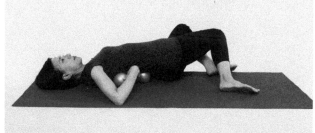
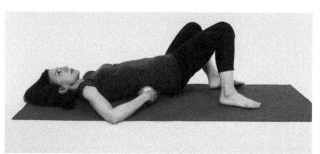
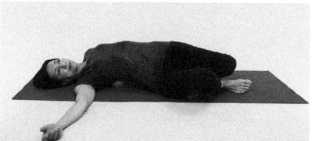

AFTER A BALL PLACEMENT

Now that you feel the benefits of the muscles being more supple, add a Whole Body Move to lengthen the lower back, improve the leg alignment and take pressure off the sciatic nerve. A nice one to try is the seated body hang over (page 63). Do you feel any more connection to the pelvis and leg joint from what we have done?

Add in the arm reaching after you lift back up on to the tip of your sitz bones using the muscle of your pelvis floor. This takes the pressure off the lower back. Is it easier after being on the ball? Do you reach easier and feel more parts of your body moving? Ask yourself these questions as you move, in order for your brain to activate new ways of reaching, breathing, and moving. If you say nothing, nothing happens.

Then come back to sitting. Notice if you sit differently. Is your head more free to go up? Are you more lifted throughout your body? Has your breathing changed?

Being able to discern differences is key. This retrains the brain–body connection to retrieve these movements during your day. Otherwise the body returns to habit. Acknowledge specific changes so you can use your body differently during your day. What you notice on the floor you can notice when you come back to stand, sit, or walk. Is your leg joint freer? Are you noticing when you hold your breath and when you're allowing your body to breathe? Are you changing out of your stuck body?

Repeat this every day. Get used to the process. It is better to do one ball placement, explore the simple directions, and feel how one change can affect your whole body, than to do dozens of mindless movements badly. Two singers can sing the same song, yet one of them moves you to tears and gives you the feeling of connection while the other is mechanical.

Don't be surprised if you go back and forth between feeling stuck and tight and then free of pain and moving freely. You will swing back and forth as your body learns a new way to move.

TROUBLESHOOTING

+ Pain while coming off the ball. It is not uncommon for beginners to like the feeling on the ball and stay there long periods of time while holding their breath stuck in one position. Going on and off the ball will solve this. Remind yourself to give in and let the weight rest. Make the *sss* sound.

+ Pain while on the ball. There should never be any pain during the ball placements. If you do have pain, there is an option to use two balls, one under each glute. Also, there is no need to lift your legs yet.

+ Feeling nothing on the ball. If you feel nothing on the ball, that's also very common. It means you are holding in a familiar habit and your brain is not sensing anything unfamiliar to notice. Use the cues. Breathing is the most likely thing people leave out and the most effective for getting changes and improvement.

CALVES ON A BENCH

Key Area: Pelvis and Leg Joint   *Star rating:* ✱

This can become your go-to at the end of a long day. Just by getting into this position, gravity will lengthen the lower back muscles, creating a sense of ease through your whole body. Add the balls, and most people feel they have found the perfect place.

Helpful Hint: Finding the right height. You should feel like your thighs are at approximately a right angle to the floor. Make sure your calves are supported from the knee down. This puts your pelvis in good alignment with the lower back. This tones up the key area of the pelvis, essential for freedom of movement. The height of the bench should not bring your feet well above your knees.

1   Check-In: Does anything stand out about the way you are sitting or lying on the floor?

2   Place your calves on a bench. If you need support for your head, place a ball behind your head and neck

   + Gradually notice how you might be holding your body in a tight position even when resting on the floor.

   + Is your pelvis tilted up or down? More to the right or to the left?

   + Use this as a time to simply let gravity and the weight of your body do the work.

3   Exhale on the *hah* sound, and slowly let your head turn on the ball.

   + Is your pelvis resting any heavier on the floor as you guide it with the cues?

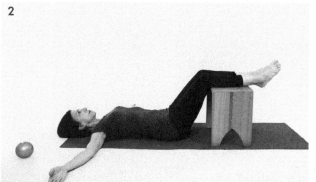

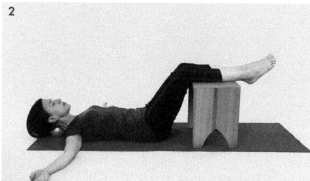

4   Remove the ball from the back of the head and neck. Slowly roll your head from right to left.

5   Gradually roll your pelvis over to the side and place the ball under the back of pelvis.

+   Allow the weight of the pelvis to lengthen the tight lower back muscles.

6   Begin to slowly roll your pelvis a little forward and back. Think of nodding your head forward and back. It's a similar movement at the other end.

7   Slowly bring your feet to the front of the bench.

+   Notice again how your legs stretch other parts of your body. Especially for those of us with sciatic pain, or stiffness in one knee or hip. Pay close attention to the differences when you move your legs in your side body. You may begin to notice one side seems to do the lion's share of the work. When you discover specific ways you move, you can begin to explore changing them. Use your tension evenly, as you bring attention to the sides. Gradually more and more will be revealed as you improve your kinesthetic sense. You don't have to work hard, just take notice of the feeling.

8   Let the legs move apart, staying aware of the different sides.

+   Make the *sss* sound and let yourself feel how gravity and the weight of your body may be making small adjustments when on the ball.

+   Slowly remove the ball and let yourself feel the weight of your body rest back on the floor.

+   Repeat this with back on the ball option 3 as well.

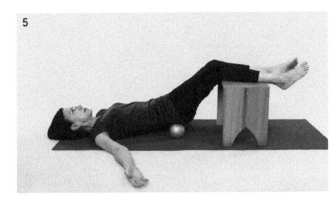

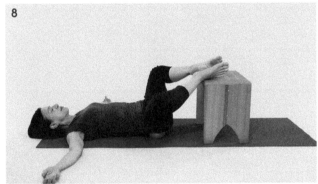

CURLING THE PELVIS

Just as we did in the Whole Body Moves, by slightly lifting your beltline, you will notice the movement in your pelvis. This is a great way to relieve lower back tightness and offer your body options. Be aware not to fight it by clenching or tucking. This is where breathing comes in. If we allow ourselves to breathe, the body cannot hold onto the habits of the past. Always allow the waist to sink again in between movements.

HEAD ON THE BALL

Key Area: Head   *Star rating:* ✳

1   Check-In, lying down:

   + Notice the space under the back of your neck, the lower back, between your shoulder blades and knees.

   + Notice where your body is touching the floor.

   + Where do you notice breathing?

2   Use one hand to lift your head and the other hand to place the ball at the base of the skull, where it meets the top of your spine. Rest on the ball. If that place does not feel good to you, then higher up the back of the head is usually easier.

3   Feel the weight on the ball and do some open-mouth breathing. Allow the weight of your head to rest.

4   Slowly begin to roll your head toward one shoulder, so slowly no one could see you moving. Repeat to the other side.

   + Remember to use the cues, like feeling the heaviness of your head and the connection to other parts.

   + Take your time. You could take a few minutes to each side.

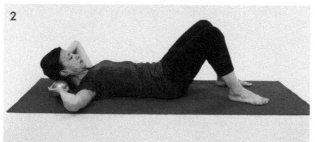

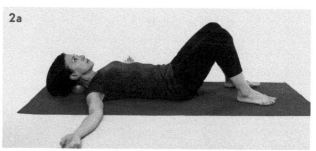

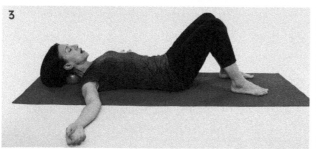

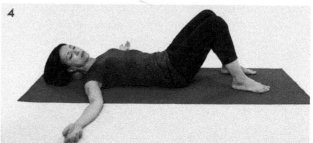

5   Return to center. Remove the ball, using one hand to support the head and the other hand to pull the ball away.

- Take the head right down to the floor; do not hold it up.

- Notice what your breathing feels like now. Do you feel changes in any other part of your body?

- Repeat two to three more times.

- When finished, slowly roll your head without the ball, freely, and feel the movement.

- Roll over onto your side and gradually come up to sitting. Be open-minded to where your head might balance in relation to the rest of your body.

- Do you find your neck lengthens?

- Do you feel any connection between your shoulders?

WHOLE BODY MOVE

Many of us may not think that the head is that important. Because the head is the heaviest part of the body, we can have great relief by allowing the head to float up as opposed to forward or back. Many of us allow our head to go wherever our habits let it. Once we are stuck in that place, it can cause pain anywhere in the back, knees, hips, and more.

After returning to a seated position, combine this ball placement with the Whole Body Move of letting the head hang forward (page 63).

- Does it feel different after using the ball?

- Do you feel more throughout your body?

- Does your breathing respond more easily?

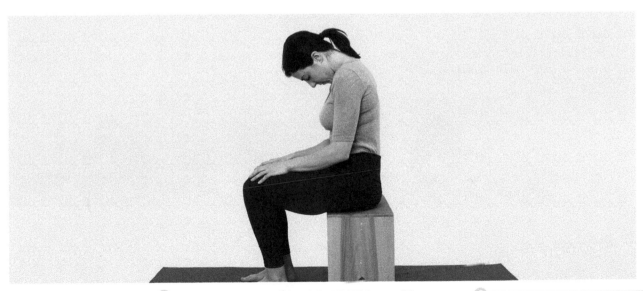

ELBOWS ON THE BALL

Star rating: ✱

1 Check-In: Begin lying down and check in.

+ Notice how your shoulders rest on the floor. Are they different?

+ Begin to make the *sss* sound as you allow gravity to help you rest your body weight.

2 Choose your tighter side if you have one. Using the ball in the opposite hand, reach across your body. Place the ball under the crook of your elbow.

3 Rest on the ball a comfortable amount of time. There should be no pain.

+ Make the *sss* sound and cue yourself to feel the weight, allowing the arm to get heavier.

+ Is there any sense of the shoulder into the side or back?

4 Reach across and remove the ball. Gradually allow the weight of the arm to rest back on the floor. Does it rest any different than before?

+ Has your breathing changed?

5 Repeat on the same side for several minutes.

6 When coming up after doing this placement on one side, notice any differences in the side of the neck.

+ Is there more distance between the shoulder and the ears on the side that had the elbow on the ball?

+ Do you notice any difference in your sides?

+ Optional: After this placement on one side, do a seated body hang over (page 54).

7 Repeat on the opposite side.

TROUBLESHOOTING

If you feel your shoulder is too stiff, you could always try placing the ball a little higher under the arm, above the elbow. Your hand does not have to touch the floor.

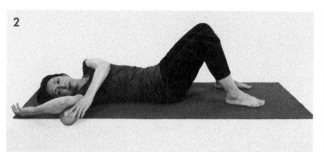

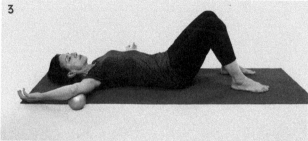

BALL BETWEEN KNEES

Star rating: ★

This is an easy placement to do when the back might need something very passive. I have done this on my side in bed while watching TV after a long day and my back was stiff as could be. Doing this in bed sometimes makes it a bit more user-friendly, and you may be more likely to make adjustments. It's great for lengthening the whole spine and improves breathing and lower back tightness.

Remember, stiffness is the lack of breath that makes it easy to hold our muscles tight, using a lot of effort during the day. As you let the leg rest on the ball, it communicates to the brain, "Stop holding," and the breath will follow. Some of us think the more we move during exercise, the better. But I have seen people stretch as a way to loosen up, but they are just doing it without much feeling. To get the benefit, they need to wait for responses.

1   Check-In: Begin lying on your side. Check in with what you notice and where you feel breathing.

2   Bend your knees at a 90-degree angle. Place the ball between your knees.

3   Notice your breathing. When you are ready, begin to slide the top knee an inch or two forward, past the bottom knee, and then return.

   + Notice if you feel this in your hips and lower back.

   + Make the *sss* sound.

4   Take the top knee behind the bottom knee. Go slowly, noticing the movement up the rest of your spine.

5   Rest in between to cue yourself before you repeat slowly. Do this as long as you feel comfortable.

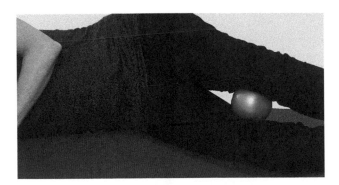
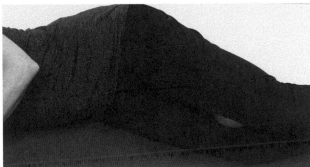

6   Take your upper body back, letting gravity open up the shoulders and rib cage. Extend your arm out to the side.

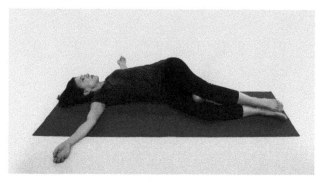

7   Gradually take the ball away and roll onto your back.

8   Repeat on the other side.

Lying on our side reflects how we sit and stand during our day. It reflects our posture. Notice:

+   Is your head forward?

+   Is your rib cage rounded back?

+   Is your pelvis tucked forward?

+   Is your bottom shoulder stiff and hurting?

After this placement, you may want to try doing a side as in Whole Body Twist (page 61). Do not force the twist, but allow the upper body to roll back.

HIPS ON TWO BALLS

Star rating: ★ ★

This placement is a different feeling than one ball and a great alternative if one ball is painful. It's a great place to use the leg joint to give relief to the lower back and to sense both sides to ease tightness on one side from sciatic pain.

1   Take a ball in each hand. Place the balls under the back of the pelvis by rolling from side to side. Rest on the balls.

2   Gradually let one knee bend out to the side. Rest and breathe, allowing the other hip to come off the ball if necessary. Keep the other leg standing, with the knee pointing to the ceiling.

3   Bring knee back up.

4   Do this several times. When the leg is open to the floor, rest.

   +   Notice what the standing knee does.

   +   Are both hips getting movement?

   +   Let gravity help you, and breathe.

5   Stretch your legs out and remove the balls.

   +   Is there a difference in your sides?

6   Repeat on the other side.

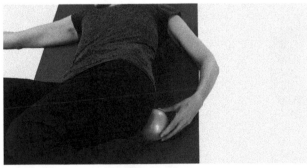

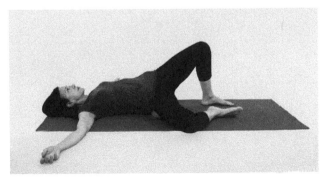

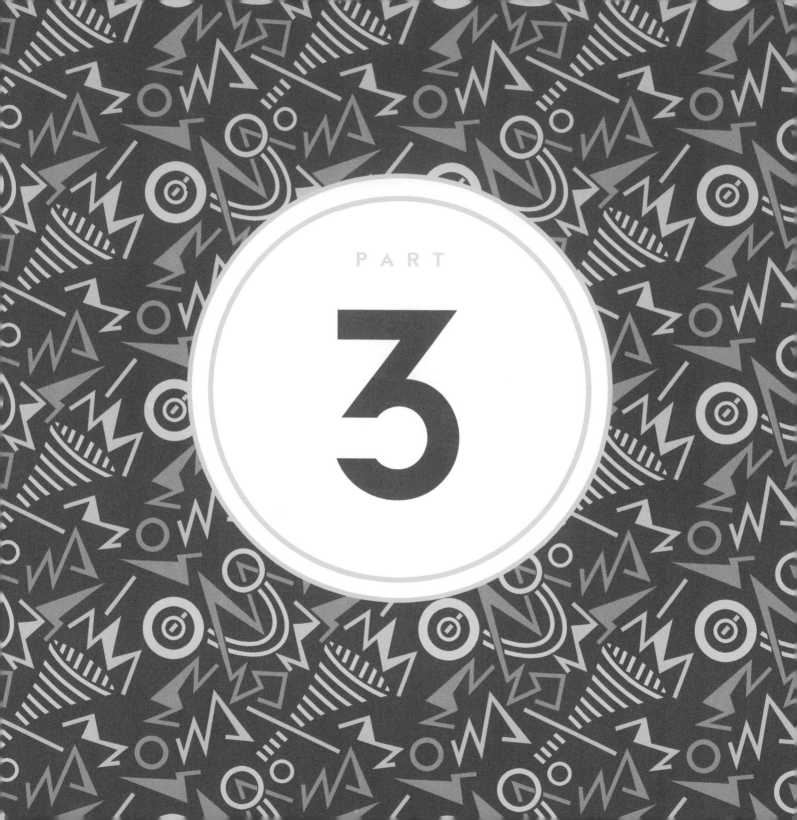

PART

3

CHAPTER SEVEN

TAKING THE METHOD WITH YOU

On-the-Go Daily Solutions

THE METHOD is using the phenomenon that through our senses our body realigns and adjusts. Our body has its own innate sense of balance. This feedback between body and brain is going on all the time. We usually don't notice it. Now we will use this ability during our day

We move away from the habits. So instead of having the same stuck ways of moving in your everyday life, we will now bring the experiences you have had on the ball with you off the ball.

It begins to work even when you are not paying attention, because you have been "inputting" new information when you are doing the Method.

I have divided this chapter into three different activity levels. The first is for those who are very inactive physically. Perhaps your job is sedentary, or you spend a lot of time driving or sitting on planes or trains. I have listed several possibilities. Then there are the more active experiences like sports, dance, or martial arts. And then your day-to-day activities, for example, simple walks, or working in your kitchen or garden. All of these are great times to use what you have learned. You will have to prod it along a bit for different activities that will enable you to use more of your body and increase strength and confidence. But it works! Your energy and creativity will improve, and it will prevent old habits from returning.

Putting your kinesthetic sense into action during your day may seem odd, but your body understands this more easily than you think. I have heard from people who take the balls with them to the gym and lie on a stretching mat after they work out. One of my students, a volleyball player, had chronic pain when she began working with me. She would go to the sideline and lie on the balls and breathe to take the pressure off her back. Your body can become stressed in an instant. But you can "unstress" in an instant as well. These skills are something you will get better and better at. We begin to know the feelings that are good and the ones that are warning us that we need to breathe, make a change. The warning signals are there, but most of us don't listen to the body.

We think our bodies are something that we control completely. If you think about that, it makes little sense. You don't control (nor would you want to) your blinking, heartbeat, healing a cut, or even every movement you make. You're more like a gardener who cultivates the soil the best they know how for their plants to grow. And because there are many factors out of our control, we need the Method. It's like anything you want to improve, you start with what you have and go from there.

Warning signals are extremely important to recognize and respond to early. They are an early warning system, and they are a byproduct of doing the Method. When it comes to our health, many people ignore warning signals and simply don't feel them.

There was a study many years ago related to migraines. The researchers discovered that the warning signals participants felt before their migraines were something another person would find alarming. But the participants had no sense of any physical changes.

The researchers began to train them with biofeedback to feel their responses ahead of time to prevent the migraine

We are doing a similar technique here. As you learn the simple process of using attention and observation, you will not accept the same holding of the breath and stuck body. Your body has options and will avoid the stuck ways of moving you were familiar with. When you do feel twinges or stiffness, which happens to anyone during stressful times, use the cues you have learned.

+ Bring attention to key areas.

+ Notice your breath and whether you begin to hold it.

+ Cue yourself based on what you notice.

+ If you find yourself slumping in your desk chair, your breathing is shallow, and you begin to feel stiff, you have options now. Or what if you are playing your favorite sports and concerned about your back? You will notice what you are doing that may be making the movements hurt with the familiar old stuck body. Do them differently. Also, everyday movements take on new meaning. Working in your kitchen, your garden, or walking down the street are all opportunities to notice how you move and just do it different. It is simple experimentation but also the body quickly tells you what is working by how you feel. The kinesthetic sense is activated simply by directing your attention to different parts of your body and your breathing.

+ Remember, you simply have to feel; you don't have to fix anything. The more parts of your body you feel, the more you will move. But be responsive. Your body is getting more and more information to help.

When you are in one position for long periods of time while you are focused on something, this can cause the body to be stuck and stressed.

Things like driving, sitting at the computer, washing dishes at the sink, playing an instrument, or standing in one place for long periods all focus our bodies in one direction, unable to move freely. Of course, this makes it difficult to breathe freely, and without the benefit of oxygen, our muscles get extremely tight. Our stress levels can rise. Our thoughts can then respond negatively to our physical feelings and then of course the cycle of pain is activated. Here are some ways to change that.

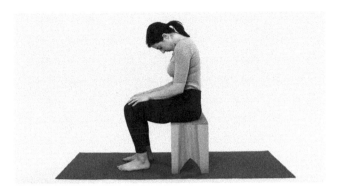

Use the weight of your head. The entire body is affected by the weight of the head, positively or negatively. Let the weight of your head bend forward and notice how much of your body responds as you "feel the weight, breathe and "then gradually lift your head back up.

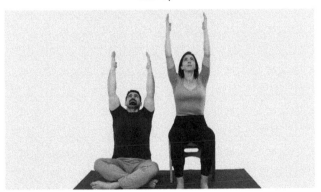

Reaching your arms up into the air. This is a quick fix that is a lifesaver. Most of us, when stuck in one position for long period,find our breathing is shallow, and our muscles get tighter and tighter. Once you get familiar with raising your arms into the air, you will feel how this lifts the key area of your ribs right off the diaphragmatic muscle in order to being much need oxygen into your body. Do this freely throughout your day.

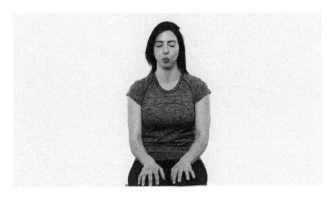

Exhale, make an sss sound. Give your body time to respond and then make the sound again.

Remember it is the combination of not just the physical restrictions, but also the thoughts we are having that add the fuel to the fire. As we learned early on, pain is the result of three things working together to keep it stuck. Your stressful thoughts, excess muscle tension, and breathing. Take a few minutes for any one or all of these quick fixes that are very specific to improve your breathing and relieve the stiffness.

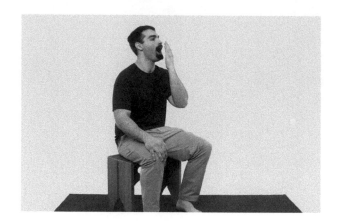

RUSHING

Rushing has the same effect on the body as being stuck in a position for long periods of time. We tend to hold our breath, and our muscles as we push from one thing to the next, which sets up the cycle of pain. Here are some common solutions. When you find yourself rushing, take a moment to notice what it is doing physically. Sometimes that will make you simply aware that you can still get a lot done, but you don't need to do it with a posture that restricts your breathing and makes your body tight and hurt.

Make an *sss* sound while you are out and about no one will even know. If you are in a city environment walking down the street, assume a lift from the top of your head and allow your movements to change. When you get to your destination, you will be more clear-headed and your energy will have improved. Use any of the directions from the previous page.

TRAVELING

If you can move around a bit, say on a train or plane, follow the directions for making the *hah* sound for ten minutes. With your hand to your mouth, no one will even know you are doing this. Then get out of your seat if possible. Your muscles will use the oxygen and stretch easily. You will be at ease and flexible when you arrive at your destination.

OPEN MOUTH BREATHING

Our bodies often feel stuck when we're in cramped places. But even in a meeting, you can stretch out your legs under the table to increase circulation.

When we hold our breath, many of us think, "If I deep breathe, that will help." Actually, it's the opposite. Exhale. Let the air out on the *sss* or *hah* sound.

Maybe you are holding your breath? Check in at times when you are stuck for long periods in one position. I have been in meetings where I simply parted my lips to allow the air to come out off and on. Your body will automatically breathe in—you don't even have to focus on it. If the air is streaming out, the diaphragmatic muscle will stretch and then naturally pull more air back into your tight body. It will also wake you up and invigorate you if you are losing focus.

SITTING FOR LONG PERIODS

If you are learning or practicing an instrument or sitting at a computer, it is common to spend long periods of time in one position. So use a timer on your phone and take breaks to get up and move around.

Reaching your arms up into the air immediately takes the pressure off the lower back and allows your diaphragmatic muscle to stretch.

Stand up, reach your arms, and let out an exhalation. Circulation is important for your back. Push your chair away from your desk and do a seated body hangover and when you come up, combine this with reaching your arms up to the ceiling. Notice how this lifts the ribs off the lower back and allows your diaphragmatic muscle to work again. When you bring the arms down you do not need to also drop the ribs down.

What you may find is when you go back to the task at hand, you are sitting differently, you can concentrate better, and more ideas flow. The body is extremely responsive with small breaks. Many of us think because we only have a minute, that's not enough. The body has very different timing.

There was a woman who got her Ph.D. studying yawning in the animal kingdom. She learned that yawning was a way to bring oxygen into the body and keep the animals alert. We sometimes need that bit of oxygen and it doesn't take much time. Use the magic of your own breath.

BEING STUCK IN BED

If you're in bed and haven't moved in a while, use the ball right there. Place the ball behind your head, wherever it feels best, and exhale. Since you are not able to move much, small movements will still work sometimes better than you think.

STANDING FOR LONG PERIODS

Many jobs require us to stand stuck in one position. This can make our backs tight and painful. Bending your knees while standing can be an easy way to take the pressure off the lower back. When most of us stand, we lock our knees along with our hips, putting all the pressure on our lower back. Gradually bend your knees while letting your lower back lengthen, then come back to standing. You may find you can then use your head to lift your ribs. Think "lengthen and lift." If you can reach your arms up to the ceiling from time to time, that will help as well.

EXERCISE AND ACTIVE HOBBIES

Now let's address enjoyable activities that require your body to move in many different directions. Activities such as exercise, dance, sports, martial arts, gardening, or taking walks are a way to increase the benefits of your improved kinesthetic sense. At this point, you will probably notice when you are holding your breath, clenching your usual areas, or having thoughts that are hindering positive cues to your body. Because these activites are happening so quickly, people will often respond, "I couldn't breathe." Our bodies are designed to breathe when they move. It is easier to move and let the body function naturally. It is habit many of us develop to hold our breath when we exercise. Think of children on a playground: do they have to remind themselves to breathe? If so there would be a lot of children passing out in playgrounds from the stress of their activities but they don't. They breathe easily because their muscles are not restricting their breathing. Simply reminding yourself that you are working harder when you hold your breath during any activity sometimes does the trick. Certainly, during any rigorous activity make an *sss* sound. Let your body do some easy Whole Body moves to let gravity bring the oxygen into your muscles. These are different than stretching. It's the cues you use, the Body Dialogue that your body is responding to.

During sports, or exercise of any kind, check in even while you are exercising. Are you locking or lengthening your muscles? Can you feel movement in key areas, do you let yourself breathe? Checking in is essential. This is simply a way for the brain to retrieve what you felt on the ball and with your whole body moves. Many of us exercise with our stuck body and don't realize it. Bodies will make choices based on

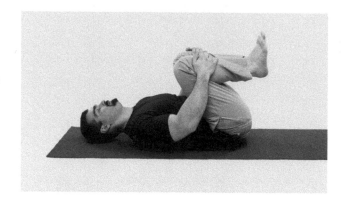

pleasure and pain. If it has options, it will go towards what feels better and you have learned the options.

Many of us when we stretch are straining, stiffening, and locking the joints. Use the Whole Body Moves directions. Incorporate them into your exercises. Any one of these activities allows you more open space to reach, bend, and move the body.

Remember, your muscles respond to your nervous system like electricity connecting all your parts. Now that you have been doing the Method, you have more feeling in all parts of your body. It's time to let your body put that into action. Notice fears or thoughts about your past that might restrict you and hold you in the cycle of pain.

Here is what you will want to focus on so that the activity you are doing is more effective and you do not end up with tight back muscles:

Notice key areas when you exercise. Common to all exercise, sports, and dance is using the key area of your pelvis and the strength of your legs. Many of us take this area for granted when it doesn't hurt. But when it does, you begin to realize that you are clenching the hips. Using the legs to support you will happen gradually if you take breaks, bend forward, and sense how gravity will help you locate new areas.

Combine the Whole Body Moves for a warm-up. Use your warm-up like your Check-In. Notice how you are moving, and gradually improve the movements and your breathing. Notice your key areas when you are warming up and exhale.

Develop your own routine. Repetition is great because you stop thinking about the movement and more about how you "do" the movement. Here are some ideas:

+ Begin gradually, in order to notice how you are moving.

+ I suggest warming up your body with seated body hang overs, whether on the floor or chair.

+ Notice your breathing.

+ Reach your arms up into the air for long side body stretches.

+ Let your head bend forward, and turn your head slowly.

+ Keep an awareness that your whole body can respond to these movements.

When doing the activity, take a few moments to use your Body Dialogue. Remember the Body Formula: weight + breath = reduction of excess muscle tension. When you are about to do a sport or an activity, can you notice how your body is shifting weight in space? Let yourself use tension for more freedom of movement. Perhaps in the past you would be concerned about your back or knee. This time, give yourself different cues, as you would when on the ball. Your brain will bring these feelings back.

Breathe. Many of us hold our breath when doing sports and exercising. You will do better to exhale and let the air out consistently. Your body will respond

DAY-TO-DAY ACTIVITIES

All day long, there are opportunities to move differently—getting up in the morning, walking through your home, sitting on a park bench—the easygoing daily things we do. If you reach for something on a top shelf, you can extend the movement through your whole body—or your thoughts may immediately set you up for failure: "Be careful, you can't reach with that side." Of course, that is giving your body an unhelpful cue.

Walking, playing with your kids, cooking, and cleaning—these can be the best times to change to move away from your habits and move differently. Chores and leisure activities both allow you time to incorporate the key areas you learned to recognize in Whole Body Moves.

When you reach, cue yourself to reach. When you

bend, think leg joints. Where's your head when you're walking? Can you sense your breathing? It's as simple as putting your Body Dialogue to work. The dialogue is happening anyway, so make it work for you.

Remember, the Body Dialogue is something that has always been with you. It is the unconscious connection between your body and brain when it comes to moving. The Miracle Ball Method brings that to a conscious level. That allows the body to adapt to new directions. We only think we can't do something because we never broke down what our thoughts were telling us. Our thoughts are also greatly influenced by others who tell us what our limitations are.

+ When you reach for something during the day, notice the rib muscles. Can you lengthen, not lock?

+ When walking, use your feet to ground you and reach your arms to the sky, like the alternative tension extension (page 85).

+ Exhale when you are walking.

+ Practice the *sss* sound with your children. My nine-year-old loved the competition of who could make it longer. He would then naturally breathe more easily. He would tell me all about his day. He was so relaxed.

+ Use the balls at home when the TV is on in the background.

+ In the kitchen, do a standing body hang over to stretch your hamstrings and prevent backache.

HELPING THE BACK AFTER A BUSY DAY

For many of us, when we finally have downtime, we want to tune out completely. That is a great time to get on the balls and breathe. Rest and recover using the Method. Once you know the Method, just getting yourself to feel the weight and allow the body to breathe does it for you.

When you have some downtime at home or in a hotel, use the easy routines you have learned for fifteen minutes to undo your busy day. It keeps your back flexible and allows your breathing to happen naturally. We recover more quickly as we get used to doing the Method.

Here are some simple solutions for those tightest areas. Use these ball placements and let yourself enjoy how strategically the balls under the key areas relieve tight back muscles, poor breathing, and more.

You can do these placements in bed before you go to sleep to "undo" your day and not wake up stiff. Each one of the routines below reminds us not to return to the stuck body and to let movement into those three

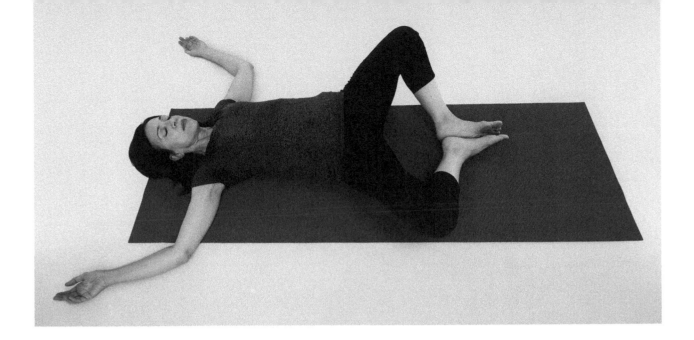

key areas. If you do this, your brain will use all the undoing day-to-day, and you will continue to improve throughout your life.

Here are a few great resting places to go to each day.

+ Lie down on the floor and place the balls under your hips. Make the *sss* sound. Let the thighs open up and let the lower back and ribs respond. Add the pelvic roll, forward and back on the ball.

+ Use the ball between the knees placement (page 80). Rest your arms over your head to arch the ribs and stretch lower back muscles. Breathe.

+ Everyone's favorite after travel or a long day is calves on a bench (page 74). Find an ottoman or coffee table to use, and gravity will do a lot of the work for you, taking the pressure off the lower back. It will also allow you to breathe easily.

COMMON IMPEDIMENTS

Here are things that will make it difficult to breathe and get out of the stuck body.

RESTRICTIVE CLOTHING

Check out your clothes. Are they rigidly holding you in place? There are many fabrics today that have a little give to them and will allow you to continue breathing. If you feel like you are in a straitjacket, your body will complain. Don't let your clothes wear you. You wear your clothes. You should be free to move, especially in key areas. If you can't breathe, it's probably the wrong attire.

HIGH HEELS

The angle of your feet as you move will, of course, change the angle of the way the rest of your body moves. Some people have no trouble with high heels, but they can pitch your pelvis forward and put more stress on your lower back. If you absolutely must wear them, take them off during the day and stretch your feet out. Walk without heels to feel your feet are getting feedback from the floor below. Do a few seated or standing body hang overs.

TIES, BELTS, AND TIGHT BRA STRAPS OR WAISTBANDS

Some of the first things people do when they get home is remove tight belts and bras or ties. Ties, tight bras, or belts all can prevent us from freely breathing and can hold us tightly in place. We don't want anything to prevent freedom of movement in the area where our diaphragmatic muscle needs to move. See if you can use belts, ties, or bras that are more moveable with your body. If you can't breathe, that is an indication it is too tight. Many of us simply get used to that feeling of stiffness until our back hurts or our body tightens up to where we cannot take it anymore.

CROSSING YOUR LEGS

Are you always crossing the same leg over the other? Do you lift the hip and shorten one side constantly? When we are sitting for long periods of time, we don't think about it. But make sure when you get up, you reach your arms and lengthen your side body, taking the pressure off the lower back. You can never be too lifted and lengthened!

WORRIES AND FEARS

"What if I make a mistake? What if I have a more serious problem?"

Since we cannot stop our thoughts, most of us don't pay too much attention to the ongoing monologue under the surface. Thoughts that we are used to are the ones we ignore.

Pay attention to them. If you begin to see a pattern of worry, hypervigilance, or always waiting for the next physical sensation to be painful, your body will

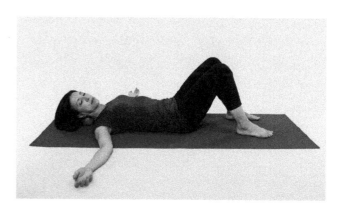

create that. Don't think you are imagining as much as creating.

Take time to notice your thoughts during the day and change the dialogue. If your thoughts are negative, I have found that doing one of the following allows our bodies to positively influence those negative thoughts.

+ Lying on the floor and checking in

+ Placing a ball behind your head

+ Make a long, extended *hah* sound.

+ Letting your jaw open gradually

+ Slowly letting your head roll

Our thoughts are part of our trained behaviors. Our body is listening. Some new cues will prevent your stuck body from returning and will give you a sense of comfort.

IS CHRONIC LOWER BACK PAIN IN MY HEAD?

Many of us think if we equate our emotions to our pain, then it's all in our head. Our bodies and our minds have a seamless connection. We have all experienced this from simple things like getting good news and your body improves and then getting stuck in a bad situation like traffic or a large bill in the mail, and very quickly your muscles might tighten, to the point of significant discomfort. Knowing this gives you the power to address your thoughts and your physical body. You do not want to ignore your thoughts or feelings but notice what you are saying to yourself in any situation and what physical responses you have. Include what happens to your breathing.

For myself, it was always more challenging to change my mood than my body. When you follow the direction in this book, you may find that as the excess muscle tension is relieved, and you are breathing easier, your thoughts improve as well. Some of the obstacles you thought were overwhelming seem not so bad at all.

CHAPTER EIGHT

COMMON QUESTIONS

as you move forward

THERE are people who have mild back problems that, once tweaked, are very easily dealt with. But for most, this process is a back-and-forth, getting relief until we take more and more of the Method with us during the day. It is something that you start out feeling, "Is this right?" and then realize, like riding a bike, that you can't imagine how it seemed so hard.

What if my pain returns?

You may begin to get relief as you start practicing the Method and then find that your discomfort returns, along with anxiety that "this is not working." Your thoughts might become very negative.

Any of us could hurt ourselves. You may have relief for a long time and then something happens. Perhaps you are playing sports, in a car accident, or simply sitting for long periods of time. One of my students remarked that she had had three previous back operations and her mother had an operation as well. But, she said, "The best thing about this Method is I never worry when my back gets tight. I know what to do."

If your pain returns or you sustain an injury, you will have to follow the same directions, get the book out again, and remind yourself of what to do. Depending on the circumstances, once the acute pain has subsided and allows you to move more easily, then begin gradually with your favorite ball placement and easygoing Whole Body Move. Begin to use your body again, letting it recover. Remember, it knows how to move. You might be surprised you recover more quickly.

Pain can make us feel frightened to move again. But you do not have to go back to that place where you had no options or solutions. Your body has learned a lot because of your direction.

Your thoughts can prevent or hinder improving more quickly. Remember, our thoughts are blended with our physical experience. Over the years, I have hurt myself doing not-so-smart things. But I didn't have the fear I had the first time or the depression when I became stuck. I want you to understand that we get better at not falling into patterns of fear and immobility. Gradually begin to move, do what you can of the Method, and you will improve. Have confidence.

What if it hurts to move?

Yes, many of us hurt when we move, especially if we are scared to death of getting a return of acute pain back. No one is as afraid as I was. People are surprised to hear that. They always say, "But you are so good at this." Yes, I am so good at it because I was so bad at it. I am not at all as good as most of my students and the responses they have.

But I worked through the fear and used my experience with the Method to guide me. I learned there are good pains and bad pains. And although I have had pain for long periods of time that left me in bed with the sheets over my head crying for painkillers, I just couldn't live like that. Those bad pains actually taught me how to move, made me stronger than I ever was before, and reshaped some of the clear weaknesses in my body.

What if it hurts where I place the ball?

There should be no pain or discomfort on the ball. If you place the ball where it hurts, especially right under the lower back, your body will not be able to continue to breathe and you will tighten up. Always adjust the ball to your body, never your body to the ball. Follow your body formula—practice reminding yourself to feel the weight of the part on the ball and notice your breathing. Most of us, when we tighten up our muscles, cannot feel the weight. The on-and-off- the-ball gives us that opportunity. So no pain on the ball; use it under another part of the body.

How long will it take?

Some of us have had a longer period of time with chronic pain, where we moved very little. Others may have had a serious accident or illness preventing them from moving. As we begin to gradually move again, the body may feel it. This can be a trigger for many to worry they are doing the wrong thing. But the body cannot improve without feeling. Sometimes you have to decide to do a little at a time and keep going. The less we move, the less we will move. The more you move, the stronger you will get. Use the Method and the advice of health professionals you trust to guide you. You should not be fearful or gloomy about moving. Going through chronic pain or healing after injuries and surgery needs an optimistic attitude. Our emotional responses to pain are understandable, but do not expect overnight changes. In fact, "expectation leads to suffering," as the Buddhists say.

Can I do other treatments while using the Method?

There is no problem with doing other treatments while

doing the Method. Use what you are learning about your body to increase your potential for healing with other treatments. Just as in any profession, there are good professionals and there are ones that don't align with your body. Your body will tell you that in how it responds.

Does pain medication interfere with the Method?

Depending on the medicine, it can be very helpful to take something to relieve the pain. It depends on exactly what your pain is from. If you are in so much fear and discomfort that you won't move, medication may help. You must discuss that with your doctor. If the medication makes you only want to stay in bed and you can't feel your body, you are probably prolonging the inevitable. Remember, we can begin to do this in bed or on the couch. Eventually, we have to move.

WHEN I wrote the first Miracle Ball Method book, my publisher gave me media training before I went on a road tour. They wanted me to discuss the Method and include my own story in three minutes or less. I had no interest and thought it was self-serving. I learned that was wrong. People wanted to know I have been there.

When I had chronic pain in my back, I did everything I was told. I used all the information, exercise, chiropractic, meditation, massage, and drugs that were available. I was determined to find a solution. But the information alone produced temporary results, if any. In the end, I was in more pain and more frustrated. The physical challenges began to combine with emotional responses. I was fearful this would never end. I felt trapped, not only physically but emotionally, as I constantly looked for more ways to relieve the pain. Eventually, I gave up.

This is when I found a teacher who just asked me to notice my own body. She directed me to notice my breathing, which I did not feel at all. Then to notice the way I was sitting, which was also puzzling to me. What did any of this have to do with my pain? And since my pain was the louder voice in the room, I was having trouble answering her.

My depression at the time—from inaction and finding no relief from any treatments—left me wide open to her suggestions. My lack of feeling at such a young age was puzzling to me. As I went through the classes, I began to notice at the end of class that I felt completely different from the beginning of class. I couldn't put my finger on it at the time, but I also couldn't ignore the fact that the responses were completely different than anything else I had tried. I felt better but I had no idea why it worked.

Somehow in that class, I was taken in a completely different direction, where my body became the canvas and I was the artist. I was—unknowingly at the time—developing an ability to know what was causing my pain by simply noticing what I felt. I realized the trap had been looking for ways to "fix" my body, not "feel" it. That became the missing link. There was no exercise, doctor, or therapist that could explain that. Does that mean anything is wrong with doctors or therapists or exercise? No. In fact, all the information you have experienced will begin to be more effective once you actually inhabit your body.

This began my journey and set me on a mission to be able to put into words what made this process work. My biggest concern with chronic pain, having been so young, was a lifetime of living with it. The thought that there was no logic to my good days and bad days was my worst nightmare. I went down every rabbit hole for hours and hours each day: using the balls, finding teachers who had studios in the back of restaurants, anyone who was taking me in a direction away from my "stuck" body.

I learned what worked and what doesn't work. Eventually, I was hired by doctors to work in hospitals and clinics. This was completely unplanned on my part. But chronic pain was something that so plagued me, and it was gone, so I had to tell others.

Back pain can be so devastating, and the message around it so restrictive, that we become trapped by the thoughts of what's next. The problem for most people is by the time they have read countless articles—articles that probably scared the life out of them and told them which way to move, breathe, and what not to do—they are so scared or confused that they spend the rest of their lives not turning right or left without worry.

This Method is an ability we all have but must relearn. Enjoy this journey. It is something that you will get better and better at throughout your lifetime.

I will leave you with this, something I tell students over the years: My job is to help you believe, like *Tinker Bell* in Peter Pan. It is not "my method," or something I'm doing to you, but something the body can do. As you follow the directions, believe in possibilities. Think of a caterpillar transforming into a butterfly. Think of dancers or athletes or small children. Your body is amazing. If humans can move, why should you be stuck? Your body knows how to do this. Let it go there. It will gradually come out of the chrysalis.

CPSIA information can be obtained
at www.ICGtesting.com
Printed in the USA
JSHW011927191121
20630JS00004B/5